WORKBOOK TO ACCOMPANY

MOSBY'S

CANADIAN
TEXTBOOK

FOR THE

SUPPORT
WORKER

THIRD CANADIAN EDITION

REVISED REPRINT

WORKBOOK TO ACCOMPANY

MOSBY'S
CANADIAN
TEXTBOOK
FOR THE
SUPPORT
WORKER

Relda T. Kelly RN, MSN
Professor Emeritus, Kankakee Community College
Kankakee, Illinois;
Parish Nurse, Wesley United Methodist Church
Bradley, Illinois

Sheila A. Sorrentino RN, PhD
Curriculum and Health Care Consultant
Anthem, Arizona

Leighann N. Remmert RN, MS
Health Occupations Instructor,
Lincolnland Technical Education Center
Lincoln, Illinois

Canadian Authors

Mary J. Wilk RN, GNC(C), BA, BScN, MN
Professor and Coordinator, Personal Support Program, Fanshawe College,
London, Ontario

Deborah Schuh RN, BN
Faculty and Program Coordinator, Personal Support Worker Program,
Durham College, Oshawa, Ontario

THIRD CANADIAN EDITION
REVISED REPRINT

ELSEVIER

ELSEVIER
MOSBY

NOTICES

The content and procedures in this book are based on information currently available. They were reviewed by instructors and practising professionals in various regions of Canada. However, agency policies and procedures may vary from the information and procedures in this book. In addition, research and new information may require changes in standards and practices. You are responsible for following the policies and procedures of your employer and the most current standards, practices, and guidelines as they relate to the safety of your work. To the fullest extent of the law, neither the Publisher nor the Author assumes any liability for any injury and/or damage to persons or property arising out of or related to any use of the material contained in this book.

The Publisher

Library and Archives Canada Cataloguing in Publication

Kelly, Relda Timmeney
    Workbook to accompany Mosby's Canadian textbook for the support worker, third Canadian edition /
Relda T. Kelly, Sheila A. Sorrentino, Leighann N. Remmert ; Canadian authors, Mary J. Wilk, Deborah Schuh. —
3rd Canadian ed., rev. reprint .

ISBN 978-1-927406-58-8

    1. Nurses' aides—Problems, exercises, etc. 2. Care of the sick—Problems, exercises, etc. I. Sorrentino, Sheila A
II. Remmert, Leighann N III. Wilk, Mary J IV. Schuh, Deborah V. Title. VI. Title: Mosby's Canadian textbook
for the support worker.

RT84.K45 2013   610.7306'98   C2013-900183-2

Vice President, Publishing: Ann Millar
Managing Editor: Roberta A. Spinosa-Millman
Developmental Editor: Joanne Sutherland
Publishing Services Manager: Debbie Vogel
Project Manager: Anitha Sivaraj
Copy Editor: Jane Clark
Proofreader: Cathy Witlox
Cover, Interior Design: Teresa McBryan
Typesetting and Assembly: GW Tech Pvt. Ltd.

Elsevier Canada
905 King Street West, 4th Floor, Toronto, ON, Canada M6K 3G9
Phone: 1-866-896-3331
Fax: 1-866-359-9534

1 2 3 4 5 16 15 14 13

Contents

Introduction

This workbook is intended to be used with *Mosby's Canadian Textbook for the Support Worker*, Third Canadian Edition. Additional resources are not required to complete the workbook exercises.

This workbook is designed as a study guide to help you apply what you have learned in each chapter of the textbook. As a supplement to this workbook, procedure checklists are featured on the Evolve Web site for *Mosby's Canadian Textbook for the Support Worker*, Third Canadian Edition. These checklists are designed to help you become more skilled at performing procedures to enhance the quality of care. Consult with your instructor for correct answers to material presented in this workbook and on the Evolve Web site's procedure checklists. The Evolve Web site for *Mosby's Canadian Textbook for the Support Worker*, Third Canadian Edition, can be accessed at http://evolve.elsevier.com/Canada/Sorrentino/SupportWorker.

As a support worker, you are an important member of the health care team. Completing the exercises in this workbook will increase your knowledge and skills. Our goal is to prepare you to provide the best possible care to your clients and to encourage you to take pride in a job well done.

CHAPTER 1

The Role of the Support Worker

TRUE OR FALSE

Circle T for true or F for false.

1. **T   F**   Most older adults have a serious illness.

2. **T   F**   Most support work with mothers and newborns takes place in the home.

3. **T   F**   Unregulated professions have no official requirements for education.

4. **T   F**   Discretion means keeping private information to yourself.

5. **T   F**   It is okay to discuss your personal problems with a client you have been working with for a long time.

6. **T   F**   The definition of *compassionate care* is treating people with respect.

7. **T   F**   Any amount of perfume can cause breathing problems for some clients.

8. **T   F**   Staff members who work together to provide health care for clients are members of the health care team.

MULTIPLE RESPONSE

From the list below, choose all of the correct answers.

9. Activities of daily living include:
   A. Bathing
   B. Toileting
   C. Feeding
   D. Personal hygiene
   E. Ambulating or transferring
   F. Taking medications

10. Support workers' responsibilities can be grouped into the following categories:
    A. Personal care
    B. Assessing and treating physical challenges
    C. Financial support
    D. Family support
    E. Legal assistance
    F. Social support
    G. Support for nurses and other professionals
    H. Housekeeping/home management

11. Which statements about support work are correct?
    A. Support work is a regulated profession.
    B. The ultimate goal of support work is to improve the person's quality of life.
    C. Support work services provided to people in their homes help them remain independent and with their families.
    D. Support work makes a difference in people's lives.
    E. Support work requires showing kindness, sensitivity, and understanding to clients.

12. The letters in the acronym *DIPPS* stand for:
    A. Identification
    B. Privacy
    C. Sincerity
    D. Preferences
    E. Discretion
    F. Personal space
    G. Independence
    H. Safety
    I. Dignity

13. To be a true professional, you should demonstrate:
    A. A positive attitude
    B. A sense of responsibility
    C. A professional appearance
    D. Discretion about client information
    E. Discretion about personal matters
    F. Acceptable speech and language

14. Practices for a professional appearance include:
    A. Following dress code policies
    B. Keeping fingernails clean and freshly polished
    C. Wearing clean stockings or socks
    D. Wearing comfortable, well-polished shoes
    E. Wearing underclothing that cannot be seen through the uniform
    F. Avoiding wearing makeup
    G. Keeping hair away from the face and off the collar
    H. Wearing mildly scented perfumes, colognes, or aftershaves
    I. Wearing a clean, well-fitting, modest uniform
    J. Wearing piercing jewellery, rings, and necklaces are made of genuine gold
    K. Covering tattoos

15. When solving problems, what things should you consider?
    A. Personal desire to solve the problem
    B. Priorities of support work
    C. Client's viewpoint
    D. Supervisor's viewpoint
    E. Scope of practice
    F. If you will be paid extra for solving the problem

16. Where should you find information about your scope of practice?
    A. Clients
    B. Supervisor
    C. Employer's policies
    D. Friends and coworkers
    E. The educational program

17. The clients you support can be grouped according to their problems, needs, and ages. Some of these groups are:
    A. Healthy older adults who live independently
    B. Mothers and newborns
    C. People with disabilities
    D. People who are in jail

E. People with medical problems
F. Athletes receiving therapy for sports injuries
G. People with mental health problems
H. People needing rehabilitation
I. Children
J. Older adults living in an assisted-living facility
K. People who have recently had a surgical procedure

MULTIPLE CHOICE

Circle the most correct answer.

18. The support worker can maintain a professional appearance by:
   A. Wearing fashionable jewellery such as a necklace or bracelet
   B. Having fingernails professionally manicured and polished
   C. Wearing a clean, pressed, and mended uniform each day
   D. Using a lightly scented perfume or aftershave

19. A support worker is considered to be:
   A. An unregulated care provider
   B. An unregulated nurse
   C. A certified support worker
   D. A regulated care provider

20. A support worker's scope of practice refers to the:
   A. Skills that the employer wants performed
   B. Amount of practice that is needed to perform a skill safely
   C. Legal extent of the role of a support worker
   D. Amount of time it takes to perform a skill

21. A primary care nurse:
   A. Performs only the basic care a client needs
   B. Cares for clients in a primary or grade school setting only
   C. Primarily works during the week and not on weekends
   D. Is responsible for the total and ongoing care of a client

22. The ultimate goal of support work is to:
   A. Make a person get better
   B. Improve the client's quality of life
   C. Never leave the client's side
   D. Do what the nurses tell you to do

23. An example of discretion would be:
   A. Speaking only to an appropriate person about a client
   B. Refraining from using the clients' names when talking about them in the lunchroom
   C. Speaking to the client's family and friends about the care the client receives
   D. Talking to your coworker about a client while you are making beds

24. Amy is a support worker who has just graduated from school. She plans on wearing her engagement ring to work once she is hired. What should you advise her about this?
   A. She will never get a job if she wears her ring.
   B. She has only a small diamond in her ring, so it would be okay to wear it.
   C. She should not wear it around her supervisor.
   D. Her ring can scratch a client, so she should not wear it while providing care.

25. Having concern for a client is:
   A. Caring
   B. Empathy
   C. Enthusiasm
   D. Respect

26. Treating the client with dignity is:
   A. Consideration
   B. Empathy
   C. Respectfulness
   D. Cheerfulness

27. Understanding your feelings, strengths, and weaknesses is:
    A. Consideration
    B. Trustworthiness
    C. Conscientiousness
    D. Self-awareness

MATCHING

Match each statement with the correct word from the right-hand column.

28. Supervises LPNs/RPNs and support workers

29. Diagnoses and treats diseases and injuries

30. Gives respiratory treatments and therapies

31. Assesses and plans for nutritional needs

32. Assists people with musculo-skeletal problems

33. Assists people with learning or retaining skills needed to perform activities of daily living

34. Treats people with speech, voice, hearing, communication, or swallowing disorders

35. Assists people with their spiritual needs

36. Helps clients and families with social and emotional issues affecting illness and recovery

A. Occupational therapist

B. Speech-language pathologist

C. Social worker

D. Dietician

E. Physician

F. Physiotherapist

G. Respiratory therapist

H. Spiritual advisor

I. Nurse

CHAPTER 2

The Canadian Health Care System

TRUE OR FALSE

Circle T for true or F for false.

1. **T** **F** Health care service delivery to First Nations and Aboriginal peoples is a provincial responsibility only.

2. **T** **F** The Canadian health care system has seen a shift in focus from home care to hospital care.

3. **T** **F** Clients are being sent home sooner after hospital procedures.

4. **T** **F** Home care enables some clients to maintain their health and independence.

5. **T** **F** The federal and provincial governments share health care costs.

6. **T** **F** Income and social status do not have an influence on health.

7. **T** **F** People can lose their medicare benefits if they are fired from a job.

8. **T** **F** Support workers provide most support services for home care.

MULTIPLE RESPONSE

From the list below, choose all of the correct answers.

9. The principles of medicare listed in the *Canada Health Act* are:
   A. Public administration
   B. Comprehensiveness
   C. Fairness to all
   D. Universality
   E. Transparency
   F. Portability
   G. Right to free speech
   H. Accessibility

10. Professional services offered within home care services include:
    A. Nursing care
    B. Laundry services
    C. Physiotherapy
    D. Occupational therapy
    E. Speech therapy
    F. Massage therapy
    G. Cooking and housekeeping services
    H. Nutrition counselling
    I. Social work
    J. Respiratory therapy

11. *Health promotion* refers to strategies that:
    A. Assist a client with legal assistance when needed
    B. Enhance or maintain a client's health
    C. Improve or sustain a client's independence

12. *Disease prevention* refers to strategies that:
    A. Prevent the occurrence of disease or injury
    B. Assist clients to improve their overall health
    C. Ensure acute-hospital funding
    D. Encourage a lifestyle of healthy eating and exercise
    E. Provide war veterans with psychological services if needed

13. Home care services today provide support to a large range of clients. These clients include:
    A. Women in labour
    B. Older adults
    C. Families with children
    D. Babies being treated in neonatal intensive care
    E. People with mental, physical, or developmental disabilities
    F. People with short-term medical conditions
    G. People with long-term medical conditions
    H. Inmates in a correctional facility
    I. Clients on telemetry (cardiac monitoring) in a coronary care unit
    J. People in the recovery, rehabilitative, or final stage of a life-ending disease

14. Examples of government policies that promote health and prevent illness are:
    A. Prenatal and parenting classes
    B. Immunization programs
    C. Same-sex marriage laws
    D. Driver's education programs
    E. Information campaigns (e.g., to reduce drinking during pregnancy, unsafe sex, and tobacco use)
    F. Age of majority legislation
    G. Efforts to improve housing, decrease poverty, monitor safe drinking water, and protect the environment

15. As a support worker, you contribute to health promotion by:
    A. Providing nonmedical care and services that can help prevent major health problems
    B. Providing end-of-life care to clients who are dying
    C. Smoking on your work breaks
    D. Placing soiled laundry immediately in the correct hamper instead of on the floor

MULTIPLE CHOICE

Circle the correct answer.

16. In 2004, Tommy Douglas was voted "The Greatest Canadian." His main contribution to Saskatchewan as health minister was to initiate:
    A. A support worker program
    B. A free food program for the people in Saskatchewan
    C. Paid 4-week vacations for everybody
    D. A medicare system

17. Private health insurance:
    A. Is available only to people who are in a low-income bracket
    B. Is illegal in Canada
    C. Must be paid for by either the client or the client's employer
    D. Is unnecessary because most people's provincial or territorial health insurance pays for all items

18. Telehealth offers health care services by providing:
    A. Phone-in prescription services to pharmacies for clients
    B. Telephone advice from nurses to people who call in
    C. In-home supportive care
    D. The telephone numbers of local doctors who are accepting clients

19. An example of a health promotion strategy is a:
    A. "Stop smoking" advertising campaign
    B. Stroke recovery program for people who have had a stroke
    C. Campaign to hire more cancer doctors in a community
    D. Program that provides hearing aids for seniors

20. It is important to identify the key determinants of a community's health because they can predict groups that:
    A. Are most likely to develop health challenges
    B. Need to be taxed more, based on their lifestyle issues
    C. Are beyond help from the government
    D. Cannot change their unhealthy behaviours

MATCHING

Match each statement below with the correct year.

21.	_____	No health insurance was available in Canada.	1961
22.	_____	Saskatchewan introduced an insurance plan to cover hospital costs.	1947
23.	_____	All provinces covered medical services provided outside hospitals.	1930
24.	_____	All provinces covered inpatient hospital care.	1972

FILL IN THE BLANK

For each of the following, mark P to indicate "professional service" or S to indicate "support service."

25. _____ Nursing care

26. _____ Physiotherapy

27. _____ Personal care

28. _____ Social work

29. _____ Assistance with activities of daily living

30. _____ Speech therapy

CHAPTER 3

Workplace Settings

TRUE OR FALSE

Circle T for true or F for false.

1. **T**　**F**　Retirement residences are financed by the government.

2. **T**　**F**　Support workers are responsible for 80% of the total hours worked by all home care workers.

3. **T**　**F**　Some hospitals hire support workers.

4. **T**　**F**　In a community day program, the support worker works independently.

5. **T**　**F**　Working in a facility requires you to do many tasks in a limited period of time.

6. **T**　**F**　Lack of privacy can lead to loss of self-esteem.

7. **T**　**F**　Another term for *acute care* is *convalescent care*.

MULTIPLE RESPONSE

From the list below, choose all of the correct answers.

8. A persistent illness is an illness that:
   A. Is ongoing
   B. May worsen over time
   C. Usually has no cure
   D. Is always fatal

9. An acute illness is described as an illness:
   A. That appears suddenly
   B. That is recurrent and untreatable
   C. That lasts a short period of time
   D. That is mild and does not require medical treatment

10. Working in home care presents issues and challenges such as:
    A. Working on your own
    B. Taking direction from different professionals
    C. Undertaking difficult tasks such as shovelling snow
    D. Maintaining professional boundaries
    E. Providing for client safety
    F. Providing for personal safety
    G. Working with other team members

11. What types of services do community day programs offer?
    A. Respite for family members
    B. Rehabilitation
    C. Counselling for people with mental illness
    D. Recreational activities
    E. Personal care services such as nail care

12. A residential facility provides care to people who:
    A. Are too young to live on their own
    B. Cannot care for themselves at home
    C. Can care for themselves independently but are too lonely to do so
    D. Require care but not acute medical care or high-level nursing care

13. The goals of long-term care are to:
    A. Provide care leading to a complete recovery or cure
    B. Maintain the clients' health and independence to the greatest extent possible
    C. Meet clients' physical, emotional, social, intellectual, and spiritual needs

14. Examples of a persistent illness include:
    A. Bone fractures
    B. Diabetes
    C. Recent urinary tract infection
    D. Multiple sclerosis
    E. Alzheimer's disease

15. Examples of acute illnesses include:
    A. Pneumonia
    B. Glaucoma
    C. Influenza
    D. Appendicitis

MULTIPLE CHOICE

Circle the correct answer.

16. Your client was admitted to an acute-care facility. Another name for this is a(n):
    A. Hospital
    B. Retirement home
    C. Outpatient facility
    D. Long-term care facility

17. Mrs. Jones receives community-based services. This means:
    A. She receives care in her community hospital
    B. She receives care after admission into a long-term care facility
    C. Her health care services are supplied outside of a facility
    D. She can receive care only in her home

18. A support worker can maintain a professional boundary with her clients by:
    A. Refusing to drive the client to a medical appointment if asked
    B. Not discussing personal problems with the client
    C. Avoiding eye contact with the client or family
    D. Giving out her home telephone number to clients

19. Often, employers will provide a newly hired worker with a written list of expected duties. Why should you ask for one if you have not received one? So you:
    A. Can find out which agency has the easiest set of duties
    B. Can negotiate which duty you want to eliminate
    C. Know what your coworkers should be doing
    D. Understand the full scope of your duties

20. Restoring a client to normal or near-normal function is the aim of which type of care?
  A. Respite care
  B. Rehabilitative care
  C. Assisted living
  D. Extended care

21. As a new graduate, you are able to demonstrate caring behaviour toward the client by:
  A. Seeking assistance before attempting a new procedure
  B. Attempting to do new treatments quickly and independently
  C. Being honest and telling the client that you have just learned this procedure
  D. Avoiding situations with clients that may be uncomfortable

MATCHING

Match the type of service with the correct description.

22. Serves people and families living with progressive and life-threatening illness

23. Provides services to people who do not need hospital care but cannot care for themselves at home

24. Provides temporary care of a person with a serious illness or disability

25. Provides services to people with immediate health issues

26. Serves people with stable conditions who may require complex equipment and care measures

27. Provides therapies and education designed to restore or improve a person's independence

28. Provides services for people with mental disorders

29. Provides care to people in their homes

  A. Respite care
  B. Home care
  C. Palliative care
  D. Acute care
  E. Long-term care
  F. Subacute care
  G. Rehabilitation
  H. Mental health

CHAPTER 4

Health, Wellness, Illness, and Disability

TRUE OR FALSE

Circle T for true or F for false.

1. T **(F)** A formal group of people who help each other is called a *social support system.* because it is an Informal

2. **(T)** F For some people, spiritual health is closely linked to religion.

3. **(T)** F Shamans are believed to use special powers to aid in the healing process.

4. T **(F)** Illness is the loss of physical or mental function. that is definition of disability

5. **(T)** F Self-image is the individual's perception of himself or herself.

6. T **(F)** Choosing athletes for a team shows discrimination against those not chosen.

7. T **(F)** It is less stressful for your client if you make all the decisions on her behalf.

8. **(T)** F Changes in sexual function greatly affect some people.

MULTIPLE RESPONSE

From the list below, choose all of the correct answers.

9. Health is defined as a state of:
   A. Making a lot of money
   B. Complete physical, mental, and social well-being
   C. Well-being in all dimensions of one's life
   D. Not just the absence of disease or infirmity

10. What are the five dimensions of health?
    A. Physical health
    B. Emotional health
    C. Financial health
    D. Social health
    E. Cognitive health
    F. Religious health
    G. Spiritual health

11. What factors contribute to physical health?
    A. Following a nutritious diet
    B. Having friends and companions
    C. Exercising regularly
    D. Living in a smoke-free environment
    E. Practising safe sex at all times
    F. Drinking alcohol moderately or not at all
    G. Having a good night's sleep
    H. Following safety practices
    I. Seeking medical attention when needed

12. How can you promote cognitive health for your clients?
    A. Encourage clients to participate in games and outings
    B. Take clients to religious services
    C. Encourage clients to read
    D. Help clients do crossword puzzles or crafts
    E. Talk with clients about community and world events
    F. Encourage clients to toilet themselves

13. What are some of the factors affecting a person's experience of illness or disability?
    A. The nature of the illness or condition
    B. Age
    C. Level of physical fitness
    D. Amount of pain and discomfort
    E. The prognosis
    F. Emotional, social, cognitive, and spiritual health
    G. Personality and ability to cope with difficulties
    H. Culture
    I. The presence or absence of emotional, social, and financial support

14. Common reactions to illness or disability are:
    A. Joy and happiness
    B. Fear and anxiety
    C. Sadness and grief
    D. Depression
    E. Increased hunger
    F. Loss of bowel or bladder control
    G. Denial
    H. Anger

15. What are some of the changes and losses associated with illness and disability?
    A. Change in routine
    B. Increase in appetite
    C. Change in work life
    D. Change in family life
    E. Change in sexual function
    F. Loss of independence
    G. Loss of dignity
    H. Change in self-image
    I. Loss of intellect

MULTIPLE CHOICE

Circle the correct answer.

16. In the past, *health* was defined as:
    A. A fit, strong body
    B. The ability to function in society
    C. The absence of disease
    D. A belief in a higher being

17. A person's culture can influence health by:
    A. Causing poor working conditions
    B. Causing an inherited disease
    C. Dictating whom the person seeks health care from
    D. Making the person strong and resilient to illness

18. Determinants of health should be viewed in relation to each other and not just individually because:
    A. They are not very important by themselves
    B. They are poorly understood by themselves
    C. Canadians do not practise good health habits
    D. Each determinant can impact the other determinants

19. Personal health practices and coping skills:
    A. Are not as important as genetics
    B. Are influenced by society and the people one is surrounded by
    C. Usually do not influence a person's ability to survive an illness
    D. Have never been linked to a healthy lifestyle

20. Holism:
    A. Considers a person's many dimensions
    B. Is not appropriate when a person has physical challenges
    C. Is a form of prejudice
    D. Is an outdated concept

MATCHING

Match the dimension of health with the correct definition.

21. __C__ Is achieved through an active, creative mind

22. __A__ Is achieved when the body is strong, fit, and free of disease

23. __B__ Is achieved through stable and satisfactory relationships

24. __E__ Results when people feel good about themselves

25. __D__ Is achieved through the belief in a purpose greater than the self

A. Physical health

B. Social health

C. Cognitive health

D. Spiritual health

E. Emotional health

CHAPTER 5

Working With Others: Teamwork, Supervision, and Delegation

TRUE OR FALSE

Circle T for true or F for false.

1. **T** **F** Only a nurse can delegate a task to you.

2. **T** **F** Registered practical nurses are not allowed to supervise support workers.

3. **T** **F** It is okay to discuss work problems with your client as long as you do not use proper names.

4. **T** **F** When you agree to perform a task, you are responsible for your own actions.

5. **T** **F** You may refuse a delegated task if you do not want to do the task.

6. **T** **F** Delegating is the same as supervising.

7. **T** **F** Support workers are allowed to perform procedures below the skin surface.

MULTIPLE RESPONSE

From the list below, choose all of the correct answers.

8. Which of the following are benefits of working on a team?
   A. Opportunities for collaboration
   B. Opportunities for communication
   C. Working with people who have a wide range of abilities, skills, and perspectives
   D. Better decision making and problem solving
   E. Dealing with conflict

9. Which of the following are usually members of the health care team in a long-term care facility?
   A. Physician
   B. Nurse
   C. Dietician
   D. Client
   E. Personal support worker
   F. Case manager
   H. Volunteer

10. When the nurse delegates a task to you in a facility, he or she is required to do which of the following?
    A. Monitor you over time to ensure you remain able to perform the task correctly and safely
    B. Assess your base of knowledge
    C. Teach you the task
    D. Make sure it is within your scope of practice
    E. Assess your performance

11. Which of the following concerns will affect delegation decisions?
    A. What is the client's condition?
    B. What are the risks involved?
    C. Can the support worker be adequately supervised?
    D. Will the support worker be required to perform the task frequently?
    E. Does the support worker want to perform the task?
    F. What tasks are included in the support worker's job description?

12. Teams in home care usually include which of the following?
    A. Family members
    B. Client
    C. Personal support worker
    D. Nurse
    E. Neighbours
    F. Case manager
    G. Social worker
    H. Physician

MULTIPLE CHOICE

Circle the correct answer.

13. When the nurse delegates a task to a support worker, who is accountable for the delegated task?
    A. The nurse
    B. The support worker
    C. The case manager
    D. The doctor

14. Which of the following is NOT one of the five rights?
    A. Right directions and communication
    B. Right supervision
    C. Right equipment
    D. Right circumstances

15. Which of the following is NOT an appropriate reason for a support worker to refuse a task? He or she:
    A. Is not trained to perform the task safely
    B. Does not know the client or resident
    C. Knows the task will require staying at work late
    D. Does not like the nurse who asked him or her to perform the task

16. Which of the following activities would be acceptable while you are at work?
    A. Making a copy of your paycheque on the photocopier
    B. Planning to eat lunch with your sister
    C. Leaving a half-hour early for a doctor's appointment
    D. None of the above

17. What are some of the challenges to working on a team?
    A. Making better decisions
    B. Having opportunities for communication
    C. Working with people who have a wide array of abilities
    D. Recognizing role boundaries

MATCHING

Match the terms with the correct definition.

18. _____ To work together toward a common goal

19. _____ The nurse on duty for that shift

20. _____ Assesses the client's needs in the community

21. _____ Transfer of function

22. _____ A function you perform for the client

23. _____ The legal right

A. Delegation

B. Task

C. Case manager

D. Collaborate

E. Charge nurse

F. Authority

Match the correct Right of Delegation with the question the support worker should ask him- or herself before performing an assigned task.

24. _____ Do I have concerns about performing the task?

25. _____ Do I feel competent in performing the task?

26. _____ Is a nurse available if the client's condition changes or if problems occur?

27. _____ Was I trained to do the task?

28. _____ Did I review the task with a nurse?

A. Right task

B. Right circumstances

C. Right person

D. Right directions and communication

E. Right supervision and evaluation

Working With Clients and Their Families

TRUE OR FALSE

Circle T for true or F for false.

1. **T**   **F**   Sympathy is the same as empathy.

2. **T**   **F**   Independence is the state of not depending on others for control.

3. **T**   **F**   When abused children become adults, they may abuse their own children.

4. **T**   **F**   You can be both a friend and a professional helper to your client.

5. **T**   **F**   Respect is showing acceptance and regard for another person.

MULTIPLE RESPONSE

From the list below, choose all of the correct answers.

6. When doing a procedure, which of the following would demonstrate the support worker is meeting the client's safety needs?
   A. Explains why a procedure needs to be done
   B. Describes how the resident in the next room handled the procedure
   C. Explains who will do the procedure
   D. Explains how the procedure will be performed
   E. Describes what sensations or feelings to expect

7. Which of the following represent different types of families you may work with?
   A. A married couple with or without children
   B. An unmarried couple living together, with or without children
   C. A widowed grandparent raising grandchildren
   D. Divorced parent living with a partner
   E. Two women or two men living together in a same-sex relationship
   F. Older parents, adult children, and grandchildren living together

8. Which of the following are factors that can influence psychosocial health?
   A. Personality
   B. Family background
   C. Environment
   D. Disease
   E. Life circumstances

9. Which of the following are elements of a professional relationship?
   A. There is a specific goal to the relationship
   B. People involved may not choose the relationship
   C. The helper is judgemental
   D. One person takes responsibility for helping the other
   E. Both people in the relationship seek to have their needs fulfilled

MULTIPLE CHOICE

Circle the correct answer.

10. Maslow's hierarchy of needs includes which of the following?
    A. Autonomy needs
    B. Competence needs
    C. Integrity needs
    D. Safety

11. Which of the following is the lowest level of basic needs as described by Maslow's theory?
    A. Physical needs
    B. Safety and security
    C. Love and belonging
    D. Self-esteem

12. Which is an indicator of a professional relationship versus a friendship?
    A. The relationship is not goal-directed
    B. The helper is non-judgemental
    C. Both people may be judgemental
    D. Behaviours are based on personal roles

13. Empathy involves:
    A. Listening and understanding
    B. The desire and actions to reduce problems
    C. Offering advice and solutions
    D. Pity

14. Dependence is the state of:
    A. Relying on others for support
    B. Relying on each other for support
    C. Not depending on others
    D. None of the above

MATCHING

Match the psychosocial task as described by Erikson's theory with the age range at which it occurs.

15. _____   Generativity versus stagnation   A.   6 to 12 years

16. _____   Initiative versus guilt   B.   1 to 3 years

17. _____   Identity versus role confusion   C.   20 to 40 years

18. _____   Integrity versus despair   D.   12 to 19 years

19. _____   Trust versus mistrust   E.   3 to 6 years

20. _____   Competence versus inferiority   F.   65+ years

21. _____   Intimacy versus isolation   G.   40 to 65 years

22. _____   Autonomy versus doubt   H.   0 to 1 year

Match one of Maslow's hierarchy of needs with each of the words or phrases.

23.   Clothing   A.   Physical

24.   Closeness   B.   Safety

25.   Experiencing one's potential   C.   Love and belonging

26.   Opinion of self   D.   Self-esteem

27.   Protection from harm   E.   Self-actualization

Match each section of the pyramid with the basic need according to Maslow

28.   Self-esteem

29.   Love and belonging

30.   Physical

31.   Self-actualization

32.   Safety

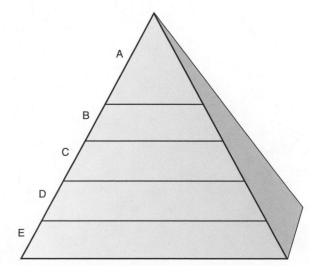

CHAPTER 7

Medical Terminology

MULTIPLE CHOICE

Circle the word in each group that is spelled correctly.

1. Slow heart rate:
   A. Bradecardia
   B. Bradycardia
   C. Bradacordia
   D. Bradicardia

2. Difficulty urinating:
   A. Dysuria
   B. Dysurya
   C. Dysuira
   D. Disuria

3. Paralysis on one side of the body:
   A. Hemyplegia
   B. Hemaplegia
   C. Hemoplega
   D. Hemiplegia

4. Opening into the ileum:
   A. Illeostomy
   B. Ileostomy
   C. Ileastoma
   D. Illiostomy

5. Blue colour or condition:
   A. Cyonosis
   B. Cyinosis
   C. Cyanosis
   D. Cianosys

6. Opening into trachea:
   A. Tracheastomy
   B. Trachiostomy
   C. Tracheostome
   D. Tracheostomy

7. Pain in a nerve:
   A. Neuralgia
   B. Neuroalgia
   C. Nourealgia
   D. Neurilegia

8. Examination of a joint with a scope:
   A. Arthoscope
   B. Arthroscopy
   C. Arethroscopy
   D. Artheroscope

9. Rapid breathing:
   A. Tachepnea
   B. Tachypinea
   C. Tachypnea
   D. Tachypnia

10. Removal of the gallbladder:
    A. Cholecystectomy
    B. Cholcystectomy
    C. Cholicystetomy
    D. Cholecistectomy

MATCHING

Match the word with the correct definition.

11.	Neuralgia	A.	Painful or difficult urination
12.	Gastrostomy	B.	Inflammation of the kidneys
13.	Cholecystectomy	C.	Bluish colour
14.	Dysuria	D.	Caused by bacteria
15.	Gastritis	E.	Study of the skin
16.	Enteritis	F.	Incision into large intestine
17.	Bacteriogenic	G.	Instrument used to examine bronchi
18.	Glossitis	H.	Inflammation of the tongue
19.	Cyanotic	I.	Nerve pain
20.	Dermatology	J.	Examination of the rectum with an instrument
21.	Oophorectomy	K.	Excision (removal) of the gallbladder
22.	Colostomy	L.	Excision (removal) of an ovary
23.	Nephritis	M.	Incision into the stomach
24.	Bronchoscope	N.	Inflammation of the stomach
25.	Proctoscopy	O.	Inflammation of the intestine

Match the prefix with the definition.

26. _____ auto-

27. _____ brady-

28. _____ circum-

29. _____ dys-

30. _____ ect-

31. _____ leuko-

32. _____ macro-

33. _____ neo-

34. _____ supra-

35. _____ uni-

A. Around

B. White

C. Self

D. Large

E. Outer, outside

F. Slow

G. Above, over

H. One

I. New

J. Bad, difficult, abnormal

Match each root word with the correct definition.

36. adeno

37. angio

38. broncho

39. cranio

40. duodeno

41. entero

42. gyneco

43. masto

44. myelo

45. pyo

A. Bronchus, bronchi

B. Duodenum

C. Women

D. Spinal cord, bone marrow

E. Pus

F. Gland

G. Mammary gland, breast

H. Intestines

I. Skull

J. Vessel

Match each suffix with the correct definition.

46. -asis

47. -genic

48. -ism

49. -oma

50. -phasia

51. -ptosis

52. -plegia

53. –megaly

54. –scopy

55. –stasis

A.   Tumour

B.   Falling, sagging, dropping down

C.   Enlargement

D.   Paralysis

E.   Examination using a scope

F.   Condition, usually abnormal

G.   Maintenance, maintaining a constant level

H.   A condition

I.   Speaking

J.   Producing, causing

Match the following phrases or terms with the correct abbreviation.

56. _____ Abdomen

57. _____ Before meals

58. _____ After meals

59. _____ With

60. _____ Cancer

61. _____ Discontinued

62. _____ Lower left quadrant

63. _____ Every day

64. _____ Range of motion

A.   c̄

B.   d/c

C.   qd

D.   pc

E.   ROM

F.   CA

G.   abd

H.   LLQ

I.   ac

Match the following abbreviations with the correct word.

65. _____   s̄   A.   Weight

66. _____   a.m.   B.   Twice a day

67. _____   CA   C.   Nothing by mouth

68. _____ H_2O D.   Three times a day

69. _____   q   E.   Height

70. _____   wt   F.   Four times a day

71. _____   ht   G.   Complete bed rest

72. _____   w/c   H.   Wheelchair

73. _____   c̄   I.   Without

74. _____   stat   J.   Every

75. _____ O_2 K.   Every night at bedtime

76. _____   abd   L.   Every other day

77. _____   CVA   M.   Morning

78. _____   bid   N.   When necessary

79. _____   CBR   O.   Right lower quadrant

80. _____   NPO   P.   Cancer

81. _____   prn   Q.   At once, immediately

82. _____   qhs   R.   Stroke, cerebral vascular accident

83. _____   ROM   S.   Left lower quadrant

84. _____   RLQ   T.   Water

85. _____   SSE   U.   Soap suds enema

86. _____   tid   V.   Oxygen

87. _____   qid   W.   Vital signs

88. _____   qod   X.   Range of motion

89. _____   LLQ   Y.   Abdomen

90. _____   VS   Z.   With

Match the following terms with the correct definition.

91. _____	Hepatomegaly	A.	Incision into the abdomen
92. _____	Hemiplegia	B.	Disease of the nervous system
93. _____	Cholecystectomy	C.	Excessive urination
94. _____	Laparotomy	D.	Deficiency of red blood cells
95. _____	Bradycardia	E.	Slow heart rate
96. _____	Neuropathy	F.	Enlarged liver
97. _____	Tachypnea	G.	Excision (removal) of the gallbladder
98. _____	Polyuria	H.	White blood cell
99. _____	Pyorrhea	I.	A disease of the brain
100. _____	Erythrocytopenia	J.	Discharge of pus
101. _____	Leukocyte	K.	Paralysis of one side of the body
102. _____	Bronchoscopy	L.	Rapid breathing
103. _____	Encephalopathy	M.	Inflammation of the mouth
104. _____	Stomatitis	N.	Examination of the bronchi using a scope

CHAPTER 8

Client Care: Planning, Processes, Reporting, and Recording

TRUE OR FALSE

The following statements apply to rules for recording. Circle T for true or F for false.

1. **T**　**F**　Write notes in pencil.

2. **T**　**F**　Include the date whenever a recording is made.

3. **T**　**F**　Make sure the writing is legible and *neat*.

4. **T**　**F**　Use any abbreviations needed to shorten an entry.

5. **T**　**F**　Use correct spelling, grammar, and punctuation.

6. **T**　**F**　Use an eraser or correction fluid if you make an error.

7. **T**　**F**　Sign all entries with your name and title as required by your agency.

8. **T**　**F**　Skip lines between entries.

9. **T**　**F**　Record what you or others did or observed.

10. **T**　**F**　Chart all care and treatments early in the shift before beginning work.

11. **T**　**F**　Record your observations, interpretations, and judgements.

12. **T**　**F**　Record in a logical and sequential manner.

13. **T**　**F**　Avoid terms with more than one meaning.

14. **T**   **F**   Paraphrase the client's words to make the meaning more understandable.

15. **T**   **F**   Chart any changes from normal or changes in the client's condition.

16. **T**   **F**   Omit unimportant information.

17. **T**   **F**   Record safety measures used in caring for the client.

18. **T**   **F**   Objective data are things a client reports that you cannot observe by using your senses.

19. **T**   **F**   Subjective data are pieces of information you can obtain about a client using your senses.

20. **T**   **F**   When you write entries in the chart, you sign your name and write your title.

MULTIPLE RESPONSE

From the list below, choose all of the correct answers.

21. What are the four senses you use to obtain information about a client?
    A. Smell
    B. Hearing
    C. Touch
    D. Instinct
    E. Sight

22. Which of the following basic observations will give you information about a client?
    A. ADLs
    B. Appetite
    C. Pain
    D. Respirations
    E. Skin condition
    F. Ability to respond

23. What basic observations can you make to determine a client's ability to respond?
    A. Can the client state his or her name, the time, the location?
    B. Does the client speak clearly?
    C. Can the client follow directions?
    D. Can the family answer questions?
    E. Is the client easy to rouse?
    F. Is the client calm, restless, or excited?

24. What observations will help to determine whether a client has normal movement?
    A. Can the client squeeze your fingers with each hand?
    B. Can the client move his or her arms and legs?
    C. Are the client's movements shaky or jerky?
    D. Does the client complain of stiff or painful joints?

25. What observations should be made about a client's respirations?
    A. Do both sides of the client's chest rise and fall with respirations?
    B. Is the client's breathing noisy?
    C. Does the client complain of difficulty breathing?
    D. Does the client complain of gas?
    E. What is the amount and colour of sputum?
    F. What is the frequency of the client's cough? Is it dry or productive?

26. What observations should be made about the skin?
    A. Is the skin pale or flushed?
    B. Is the skin moist or dry?
    C. Is the skin intact?
    D. Are bruises present? Where?
    E. Is the abdomen firm or soft?
    F. Does the client complain of itching?

27. What observations are important to determine how the bowels and bladder are functioning?
    A. Amount, colour, and consistency of stool
    B. Colour of the lips and nail beds
    C. Frequency of bowel movements
    D. Pain or difficulty urinating
    E. Client's control of the passage of urine
    F. Frequency of urination

28. When reporting to the nurse, you should do which of the following?
    A. Report what you observed and did yourself
    B. Report what other support workers did
    C. Report any changes in the client's condition.
    D. Report promptly, thoroughly, and accurately
    E. Report only at the end of your shift

MULTIPLE CHOICE

Circle the correct answer.

29. Which of these is not a rule of communication?
    A. Use words that have only one meaning.
    B. Give a very detailed and lengthy explanation.
    C. Be specific and concise when giving information.
    D. Organize information in a logical manner.

30. What information is not included on the graphic sheet?
    A. Temperature, pulse, respirations
    B. Bowel sounds
    C. Height and weight
    D. Bowel movements

31. The Kardex is a:
    A. Part of the medical record (chart)
    B. Sheet used to record measurements or observations

C. Written description of the nursing care given
D. Summary of treatments, diagnoses, and routine care measures

32. Which of these is a question about an activity of daily living?
    A. Can the client perform personal care without help?
    B. How much food on the tray did the client eat?
    C. What is the frequency of the client's bowel movements?
    D. Can the client move his or her arms and legs?

33. The purpose of a team meeting is to:
    A. Identify the medical diagnosis
    B. Develop or revise a client's nursing care plan for effective care
    C. Share the end-of-shift report
    D. Chart the day-to-day care of the client

FILL IN THE BLANK

The following words or phrases are either subjective (S) or objective (O) data. Fill in the blank with either an S or an O.

34. _____ Sleepy

35. _____ Chest pain

36. _____ Cool skin

37. _____ Bruises

38. _____ Difficulty breathing

39. _____ Gas pain

40. _____ Pain when urinating

41. _____ Productive cough

42. _____ Breath has a fruity odour

43. _____ Rapid pulse and shallow breathing

44. _____ Mr. Khan states that he is cold

45. _____ Mary has red hair

46. _____ Mrs. Smith says she has pain in her right shoulder

47. _____ Temperature 37.6°C (99.6°F), pulse 72, respirations 16

48. _____ Mr. Kallio ate all of his breakfast

49. _____ Mrs. Foster says she is anxious about having surgery

MATCHING

Match the following descriptions with one of the key terms related to communication.

50. _____ Identification of a disease or condition by a doctor

51. _____ Determining if the goals in the care plan have been met

52. _____ Statement describing a health problem that can be treated by nursing measures

53. _____ Written guide that gives direction about the care and services a client should receive

54. _____ Method used by nurses to plan and deliver nursing care

55. _____ Action taken by a nursing team member to help the client reach a goal

A. Nursing care plan

B. Nursing diagnosis

C. Nursing intervention

D. Care planning process

E. Medical diagnosis

F. Evaluation

Match the following time with the corresponding time using the 24-hour clock

56. _____   8:45 a.m.   A.   0030 hr

57. _____   4:00 p.m.   B.   2400 hr

58. _____   11:59 p.m.   C.   2200 hr

59. _____   12:30 a.m.   D.   0630 hr

60. _____   9:50 p.m.   E.   1930 hr

61. _____   midnight   F.   1530 hr

62. _____   6:30 a.m.   G.   0845 hr

63. _____   10:00 p.m.   H.   2359 hr

64. _____   1:30 p.m.   I.   1445 hr

65. _____   7:30 p.m.   J.   1330 hr

66. _____   3:30 p.m.   K.   2150 hr

67. _____   2:45 p.m.   L.   1600 hr

CHAPTER 9

Managing Stress, Time, and Problems

TRUE OR FALSE

Circle T for true or F for false.

1. **T** **F** Stressors over a short period of time can cause a persistent illness.

2. **T** **F** You should set weekly goals for yourself.

3. **T** **F** Getting a promotion can cause stress.

4. **T** **F** A child usually shows different signs of stress than an adult.

5. **T** **F** Time management is essential to reducing stress.

6. **T** **F** There is no point in planning your work a day ahead since things change when you get to work.

7. **T** **F** You don't need to report a conflict with a client if it is resolved.

8. **T** **F** In a home care setting, you must plan your time so you can be on time for the next client.

9. **T** **F** Older adults are less able to cope with stress.

10. **T** **F** All stress is bad for your well-being.

MULTIPLE RESPONSE

From the list below, choose all of the correct answers.

11. Which of the following strategies can help you manage stress in your life?
    A. Think positively.
    B. Develop self-awareness.
    C. Ask for help and support.
    D. Be aggressive.
    E. Practise calming exercises.

12. Which of the following can help you save time and stay organized?
    A. Identify priorities.
    B. Set goals.
    C. Multi-task.
    D. Make daily plans.
    E. Make a weekly plan.

13. Which of the following strategies can you use to manage conflict at work?
    A. Identify and solve problems before they become major issues.
    B. Explain the situation to a coworker and ask for advice.
    C. Arrange a private meeting with the person with whom you have a conflict.
    D. Explain the problem to the person, focusing on the facts, not on the person.
    E. Listen to the other person's response without interrupting.

14. Which of the following can be physical signs of stress?
    A. Rapid pulse
    B. Rapid respirations
    C. Decreased blood pressure
    D. Slow speech
    E. Difficulty swallowing
    F. Difficulty sleeping

15. Emotional and behavioural signs of stress can include which of the following?
    A. Anxiety
    B. Depression
    C. Anger
    D. Increased self-esteem
    E. Poor concentration
    F. Drinking

16. Which of the following represent the acronym *SMART* when referring to goals?
    A. Specific
    B. Simple
    C. Measurable
    D. Manageable
    E. Achievable
    F. Reliable
    G. Realistic
    H. Timely
    I. Team

MULTIPLE CHOICE

Circle the correct answer.

17. Which of the following defines *anxiety*?
    A. An unconscious reaction that blocks unpleasant feelings
    B. A state of exhaustion
    C. An event that causes stress
    D. A vague, uneasy feeling

18. Which of the following defines *projection*?
    A. Assigning one's feelings to someone or something else
    B. Acting in a way that is opposite to what you feel
    C. Reverting or moving back to earlier behaviours
    D. Changing an emotion into a physical reaction

19. Which of the following is a physical sign of stress?
    A. Forgetfulness
    B. Fear
    C. Sweaty palms
    D. Anger

20. Which strategy will help you manage stress?
    A. Sleeping more
    B. Developing self-awareness
    C. Trying to manage everything yourself
    D. None of the above

21. You may encounter conflict with the client's family because:
    A. They are just being difficult
    B. They want to be in control
    C. They do not understand the nursing care plan
    D. They do not like you

MATCHING

Match the term with the definition.

22. _____   Giving an acceptable reason or excuse for one's behaviour or actions

23. _____   Transferring one's behaviour or emotions from one person, place, or thing to another

24. _____   Expressing or changing an emotion into a physical symptom

25. _____   Keeping unpleasant or painful thoughts or experiences from the conscious mind

26. _____   Directing emotions toward another person or thing that seems safe rather than toward the person or thing that is the source of the emotions

27. _____   Refusing to face or accept something that is unpleasant

28. _____   Acting in a way that is opposite to what one truly feels

29. _____   Retreating or moving back to an earlier time or condition

A.   Conversion

B.   Denial

C.   Displacement

D.   Projection

E.   Regression

F.   Rationalization

G.   Repression

H.   Reaction formation

CHAPTER 10

Ethics

TRUE OR FALSE

Circle T for true or F for false.

1. **T** **F** Support workers have a formal code of ethics.

2. **T** **F** Clients can decide what kind of treatments they want.

3. **T** **F** You can uphold the principle of justice by being concerned about all clients.

4. **T** **F** It is okay to talk about a client in the locker room.

5. **T** **F** There is nothing wrong with accepting a dinner invitation from a member of a client's family.

6. **T** **F** A support worker is free to discuss a client's progress or treatment with a close family member.

7. **T** **F** You should not take sides with a client against a family member.

8. **T** **F** Becoming personally involved with clients or their families may prevent you from providing non-judgemental care.

MULTIPLE RESPONSE

From the list below, choose all of the correct answers.

9. Ethics refers to:
   A. Laws that govern our community
   B. Beliefs that determine what is good or bad
   C. Guidelines that help us to decide what is right or wrong
   D. Moral principles or values that guide our choices

10. Which points should be included in a sample code of ethics for support workers?
    A. Provide high-quality personal care and support services.
    B. Provide compassionate care to paying clients only.
    C. Value the dignity of all clients.
    D. Respect clients' choices about how they receive or participate in their care.
    E. Respect clients' rights to privacy and confidentiality.
    F. Do not misuse the support worker's position of trust
    G. Be reliable most of the time.
    H. Promote and maintain clients' safety

11. The four basic principles of health care ethics are:
    A. Autonomy
    B. Honesty
    C. Justice
    D. Beneficence
    E. Maleficence
    F. Nonmaleficence

12. Which of the following points will *correctly* assist you to decide on a course of action when faced with an ethical dilemma involving a client?
    A. Consider the five principles of health care ethics.
    B. Collect as much information about the situation as possible.
    C. Consider a few of your available options.
    D. Determine if the action provides you with a short-term or long-term benefit.
    E. Consider if the action will treat the client justly and fairly.
    F. Decide if the action can cause harm or increase the risk of harm to the client.
    G. Consider the client's wishes and preferences before deciding.

MULTIPLE CHOICE

Circle the correct answer.

13. Ethics is:
    A. Concerned with what is right and wrong behaviour
    B. Making bad judgements before knowing the facts
    C. Deciding whether a situation is right or wrong based on your own life experiences
    D. A law telling you what you can and cannot do

14. You ask Ms. Burton if she is ready to get dressed. She says, "I would like to wait until after breakfast." She is exercising her right to:
    A. Privacy
    B. Freedom from abuse, mistreatment, and neglect
    C. Personal choice
    D. Be free from restraint

15. Ms. Burton will not consent to a physical examination. She is exercising her right to:
    A. Personal choice
    B. Privacy
    C. Quality of life
    D. Refuse treatment

16. Ms. Burton continues to refuse to take a shower. Which is true?
    A. The staff can force Ms. Burton to shower.
    B. Ms. Burton's family should force her to shower.
    C. The staff needs to first find out why she refuses to shower.
    D. The staff should immediately report Ms. Burton's refusal to the supervisor.

17. *Work ethics* refers to:
    A. Trusting others with information
    B. Being polite and considerate
    C. Behaviour in the workplace
    D. Right and wrong conduct

18. An example of just treatment includes:
    A. Treating everybody with fairness
    B. Talking about others in the cafeteria
    C. Avoiding a client whose lifestyle you do not approve of
    D. Lying about someone to avoid embarrassment

MATCHING

Match each definition with the correct term.

19. Seeking to do no harm

20. Doing or promoting good

21. Abuse

22. All people should be treated in a fair manner

23. Accidental injury or negligence

24. Having free choice

A. Autonomy

B. Justice

C. Beneficence

D. Intentional harm

E. Nonmaleficence

F. Unintentional harm

CHAPTER 11

Legislation: The Client's Rights and Your Rights

TRUE OR FALSE

Circle T for true or F for false.

1. T   F   Employment standards and legislation protect you from harassment.

2. T   F   Libel is making false statements in print.

3. T   F   The unnecessary use of restraints is false imprisonment.

4. T   F   Civil laws deal with relationships between people.

5. T   F   A physician can ask you to obtain a consent from a client.

6. T   F   You may refuse to do something beyond your scope of practice.

7. T   F   A common act of courtesy is one way to respect a client's dignity.

8. T   F   It is okay to open a client's mail in case it contains upsetting news.

9. T   F   Respecting a client's dignity can encourage independence.

10. T   F   It is important to tell the nurse when you leave and return to the unit for meals and breaks.

11. T   F   Human rights legislation protects against harassment.

MULTIPLE RESPONSE

From the list below, choose all of the correct answers.

12. Basic human rights in Canada include:
    A. The right to equality before and under the law, without discrimination based on race, ethnic origin, colour, religion, sex, age, or disability
    B. Freedom of action
    C. Freedom of thought, belief, opinion, and expression
    D. Freedom of peaceful assembly and association
    E. The right to drive
    F. The right to vote
    G. The right to enter, remain in, and leave Canada
    H. The right for illegal immigrants to stay in Canada
    I. The right to life, liberty, and security of the person
    J. Freedom of conscience and religion

13. Most long-term care facilities have policies that recognize that residents have the following rights:
    A. To be treated with dignity and respect
    B. To live in a safe and clean environment
    C. To be properly sheltered, clothed, groomed, and cared for
    D. To keep and display personal possessions, pictures, and furnishings in their rooms
    E. To have family present 24 hours a day if the person is dying
    F. To have hairdressing and barber services provided free of charge
    G. To be free from abuse
    H. To discuss problems or suggest changes to any aspect of the services provided to them
    I. To privacy and confidentiality
    J. To give or withhold informed consent
    K. To a autonomy (the right to make decisions)

14. How can you show respect to your clients?
    A. Be courteous
    B. Respect the person's belongings and property
    C. Avoid eye contact
    D. Try to do as much as you can for the client
    E. Assist with personal care and grooming whenever—and only if—necessary
    F. Be patient
    G. Listen attentively
    H. Address an adult by title and last name, unless the person tells you to do otherwise
    I. Never scold, laugh at, or embarrass the person

15. Informed consent for a treatment should include knowledge about:
    A. Potential risks and side effects of the treatment
    B. The reason for the treatment or service
    C. How the treatment will be done
    D. Who will be doing the treatment
    E. The expected outcomes
    F. What will be done during the treatment
    G. Other treatment options
    H. The health care worker's opinions of the treatment
    I. The likely consequences of not having the treatment

MULTIPLE CHOICE

Circle the correct answer.

16. If a client has different values or standards from yours, you should:
    A. Respect the client as an individual
    B. Refuse to care for the client
    C. Firmly tell the client what your values are
    D. Discuss the client's beliefs with others at work or at home

17. If you are asked to obtain a client's signature on an informed consent, you should:
    A. Make sure the client is mentally competent
    B. Refuse because this is not a support worker's responsibility
    C. Ask a family member to witness the signature
    D. Call the doctor to witness the signature

18. If a client refuses treatment, what action should be taken by the health care facility?
    A. Give the treatment as ordered
    B. Honour the request and discontinue the treatment
    C. Find out what the client is refusing and why
    D. Tell the family that the client must be removed from the facility

19. A client tells you he is upset because he believes his treatment was done incorrectly yesterday. Your action is based on which of the following?
    A. He has a right to voice his concerns and to have the facility try to correct the matter.
    B. You know the treatment was done correctly.
    C. He complains constantly, so everyone ignores his concerns and questions.
    D. He is confused and forgets what was done yesterday.

20. What rights do clients have?
    A. They may discuss concerns and offer ideas.
    B. They may take part in social, cultural, religious, and community activities.
    C. They may receive support and reassurance from family members and friends.
    D. All of the above.

21. What action by the support worker protects the client's right to personal possessions?
    A. Throwing away old cards, letters, and magazines to tidy the unit
    B. Re-arranging personal items so they are more decorative
    C. Getting the client's permission to look for an item in the closet
    D. Taking a piece of candy from the client's candy dish when he or she is not present

22. An *advance directive* is:
    A. The care plan
    B. An order not to resuscitate the client
    C. A document stating the client's wishes about health care when he or she is unable to make the decision independently
    D. A document stating the client's wishes about his or her end-of-life care

23. A legal right is something that a person:
    A. Must earn by getting a job
    B. Must be a certain age to get
    C. Is entitled to in Canada
    D. Can get by applying for it from the government

24. When a client complains to you about the home care agency's policies, you should:
    A. Defend the agency and the policy
    B. Check the client's mental status on the Kardex
    C. Inform your supervisor of the complaint
    D. Act interested and record it in your notepad

25. A living will addresses the client's wishes about:
    A. Preferences about the care used to sustain the client's life
    B. Care and guardianship of the client's young children
    C. Having a tree planted in the client's name
    D. Who will receive the client's assets and property once the client has died

26. Who is responsible for job safety in a long-term care facility?
    A. The clients
    B. The maintenance staff who repair broken equipment
    C. Both employers and employees
    D. The provincial minister of health

MATCHING

From the list provided, choose the word that best fills in the blank in each statement.

27. If a client complains of chest pain and you do not report it to your supervisor, this is a _____ act.

28. Discussing a client's treatment with your best friend invades the client's _____.

29. In order to protect the client's right to privacy, the client's body must not be needlessly _____.

30. Consent is needed for _____ to observe the client's care.

31. The client has the right to _____ and _____ mail without interference.

32. Information about the client's _____, _____, and condition is kept confidential.

33. An individual has failed to act in a reasonable and careful manner and caused harm to the person or the person's property. This is a tort known as _____.

34. A support worker opens a client's mail and reads it. This is a tort known as _____.

A. Care; treatment

B. Privacy

C. Negligent

D. Negligence

E. Invasion of privacy

F. Others

G. Send; receive

H. Exposed (or uncovered)

From the list provided, choose the word that best fills in the blank in each statement.

35. After her morning care is completed, a client wants to do activities. The support worker does not allow the client to go. This is a tort known as _____.

36. A living will addresses the client's wishes about his _____ when he is at a point when he cannot speak for himself.

37. While cleaning a client's dentures, the support worker drops and breaks them. This is a tort known as _____.

38. Instead of allowing the client a choice, the support worker tells the client that she will get a shower whether or not she wants one. This is a tort known as _____.

39. An individual makes defamatory statements about another person. This is a tort known as _____.

40. A support worker talks to employees from other departments about a client. This is a tort known as _____.

41. Your best protection against charges of negligence is _____ every procedure.

42. The client is allowed to visit family and friends in _____.

A. Slander

B. Assault

C. Documenting (or recording)

D. Private

E. Negligence

F. False imprisonment

G. Care

H. Invasion of privacy

From the list provided, choose the word that best fills in the blank in each statement.

43. A client pressed the call bell 20 minutes ago. When no one responds, he tries to go to the bathroom alone, slips and falls, and breaks a hip.

This is a tort known as _____.

44. An individual has injured the name and reputation of a person by making false statements to a third person. This is a tort known as _____.

45. An individual attempts or threatens to touch another person's body without the person's consent. This is a tort known as

_____.

46. An individual touches another person's body without the person's consent. This is a tort known as

_____.

47. An individual exposes the private affairs of another person to a third person. This is a tort known as

_____.

48. An individual restrains or restricts another person's freedom of movement without a physician's order. This is a tort

known as _____.

49. A worker causing harm to a person deliberately is

called an _____ act.

50. A will addresses the client's wishing about personal

_____.

A.   Invasion of privacy

B.   Intentional

C.   Negligence

D.   False imprisonment

E.   Slander

F.   Assault

G.   Battery

H.   Property

Match the words and definitions.

51. _____   What you should or should not do

52. _____   Having free choice

53. _____   Legally responsible

54. _____   Wrongful act committed against a person or a person's property

55. _____   A body of laws

56. _____   Failing to act in a competent manner

57. _____   Touching a person's body without consent

58. _____   Injuring the reputation of a person by making false statements

59. _____   Specific law

60. _____   Something to which a person is justly entitled

A.   Right

B.   Legislation

C.   Liable

D.   Negligence

E.   Ethics

F.   Act

G.   Autonomy

H.   Battery

I.   Defamation

J.   Tort

CHAPTER 12

Caring About Culture and Diversity

TRUE OR FALSE

Circle T for true or F for false.

1. **T   F**   People of all cultures are comfortable with physical touch.

2. **T   F**   In Western cultures, personal space is about 120 cm (4 feet).

3. **T   F**   Silence can be a sign of respect in some cultures.

4. **T   F**   Some children rebel against the culture of their parents.

5. **T   F**   You should never try to convert your clients to your own belief system.

6. **T   F**   All folk remedies are harmless.

7. **T   F**   Discrimination leads to prejudice.

8. **T   F**   In Vietnam, men do not shake women's hands.

9. **T   F**   In Asian cultures, eye contact can be considered disrespectful.

10. **T   F**   Asking about your client's beliefs and values will help him or her feel valued and respected.

MULTIPLE RESPONSE

From the list below, choose all of the correct answers.

11. Culture affects a person's beliefs and behaviour in the areas of:
    A. Communication
    B. Receiving wages and earnings
    C. Family and social organization
    D. Religion and worship
    E. Health care practices and reactions to illness
    F. Body shape and intelligence

12. Non-verbal cues can include:
    A. Touch
    B. Personal space
    C. Using kind words when speaking
    D. Eye contact
    E. Facial expressions

13. Many facial expressions that convey emotions are universal; some of them are:
    A. Anger
    B. Pain
    C. Surprise
    D. Embarrassment
    E. Happiness

14. An extended family may include:
    A. Parents
    B. Grandparents
    C. Neighbours
    D. Friends
    E. Children
    F. Aunts
    G. Cousins

15. Religions may promote beliefs and practices related to:
    A. Daily living habits
    B. Behaviours
    C. Relationships with others
    D. Diet
    E. Healing
    F. Days of worship
    G. Birth and birth control
    H. Medicine
    I. Death

16. To be tolerant and understanding of others, you need to understand:
    A. Everything about other cultures
    B. How your culture influences you
    C. How culture influences clients' behaviours and attitudes
    D. All people are the same
    E. Each client is unique, and individuals may not follow every belief and practice of their culture or religion

17. When you communicate with people who don't speak your language, you should:
    A. Convey comfort by the tone of your voice and with your body language
    B. Speak loudly or shout your message
    C. Speak slowly and distinctly
    D. Keep messages short and simple
    E. Be alert for words the client seems to understand
    F. Use gestures and pictures
    G. Repeat the message using the same words so they understand you
    H. Use slang terms since these are usually understood
    I. Be certain the client understands what is going to happen and consents before you begin a procedure
    J. Learn a few useful phrases in the client's language

MULTIPLE CHOICE

Circle the correct answer.

18. People of Asian background may conceal negative emotions with a:
    A. Laugh
    B. Smile
    C. Frown
    D. Stare

19. Sam and Chris are a couple who share parenting responsibilities for two children. Sam is the parent of one of the children, but both Sam and Chris are the legal parents of the other child. This is an example of a

    _____ family.
    A. Blended
    B. Nuclear
    C. Single-parent
    D. Separated

20. Culture is considered to be more than just a person's ethnicity because:
    A. It can refer to characteristics learned by living in any group (e.g., a group of college students)
    B. Most Canadians do not have an ethnic background
    C. Ethnicity has nothing to do with culture
    D. There is no such thing as ethnicity

21. Jim is a homosexual man who was recently beaten up after leaving a gay bar with a friend. This is an example of:
    A. Racism
    B. Agism
    C. Homophobia
    D. Sexism

22. Tony's parents came to Canada from Italy when Tony was 3 years old. He is expected to marry someone who is also of Italian descent. However, Tony is seriously dating someone from an Asian background. This situation is an example of:
    A. Cultural stereotyping
    B. Cultural conflict
    C. Ethnic cleansing
    D. Ethnic identity

23. A traditional nuclear family consists of a:
    A. Mother, father, and children
    B. Mother, father, children, and grandparents
    C. Mother and children
    D. Father, father, and children

24. Gayle has refused to take her prescribed blood pressure medication because of her religious faith. However, her family would like you to "sneak" her pills into her by grinding them and adding them to her food. Your best response to her family would be:
    A. "If you want me to do this, it'll cost you money!"
    B. "Are you kidding? I could get fired for this!"
    C. "It would be wrong for me to go against a client's wishes."
    D. "Why don't you do it while I leave the room?"

25. Mrs. Jing, who is a Buddhist, would like to pray and has asked if you could pray with her. You practise a different faith. What should you say to her request?
    A. "I'm not a member of that religion. Let me find someone who is."
    B. "No way. I don't believe in any of that."
    C. "I am not allowed to pray with clients."
    D. "I'll stay with you and support you while you pray."

26. Mr. Jones has asked for a male support worker as his religion states that it is improper to be touched by a female other than his wife. There are no male support workers working that day. How should you handle this situation?
    A. Speak to your supervisor about the situation immediately
    B. Tell Mr. Jones that you are the only one available and that he should be happy to get any care at all
    C. Care for him but wear gloves to avoid skin-to-skin contact
    D. Tell him to do his own care

MATCHING

Match the terms and definitions.

27. _____   Characteristics of a group of people

28. _____   An overly simple or exaggerated impression of a person

29. _____   The unfair treatment of people based on their group membership

30. _____   The area immediately around one's body

31. _____   Groups of people who share similar physical features

32. _____   Groups of people who share a common history

33. _____   An attitude that judges a person based on his or her membership in a group

A.   Race

B.   Prejudice

C.   Ethnic group

D.   Culture

E.   Personal space

F.   Stereotype

G.   Discrimination

CHAPTER 13

Interpersonal Communication

TRUE OR FALSE

Circle T for true or F for false.

1. **T F** The same word can mean something different to two people.

2. **T F** Touch is not a type of communication.

3. **T F** When paraphrasing, expand on the message and use more words to ensure you understand.

4. **T F** Non-verbal clues often reflect a client's true feelings.

5. **T F** Most older clients are not aware of your body language.

6. **T F** Closed questions can be answered with "yes" or "no."

7. **T F** Focusing is useful when a client rambles.

8. **T F** Short sentences are more clearly understood.

9. **T F** It is not important to be at eye level when communicating.

10. **T F** Using pet names such as "dear" can improve communication.

11. **T F** Assertive communication is the same as aggressive communication.

12. **T F** You can use open-ended questions to start a conversation.

13. **T F** Gestures, facial expressions, posture, body movements, touch, and appearance are ways of communicating without words.

14. **T F** When you hold a client's hand or touch the shoulder to convey caring or warmth, you are using verbal communication.

15. **T F** A client who denies having pain but protects a body part by lying in a certain way is using body language to communicate.

16. **T   F**   When a support worker frowns or wrinkles the nose because the client has body odour, the support worker is sending a message through body language.

17. **T   F**   A support worker telling a client "Don't worry" or "Everything will be okay" may be a barrier to effective communication.

MULTIPLE RESPONSE

From the list below, choose all of the correct answers.

18. Body language includes which of the following?
    A.   Appearance
    B.   Facial expressions
    C.   Posture
    D.   Tone of voice
    E.   Eye contact
    F.   Gestures

19. To effectively communicate with words, you need to:
    A.   Choose words carefully
    B.   Pretend to understand
    C.   Ask one question at a time
    D.   Speak clearly, quickly, and distinctly
    E.   Control your volume and tone of voice
    F.   Be brief and concise
    G.   Determine understanding
    H.   Use simple, everyday language

20. Guidelines for active listening include:
    A.   Making eye contact
    B.   Facing the client
    C.   Responding to the client
    D.   Leaning toward the client

21. What are some of the barriers to good communication?
    A.   Hearing impairment
    B.   Vision impairment
    C.   Nervous system disorders
    D.   Too much privacy

E.   Cultural differences
F.   Loud noises
G.   Distractions

22. Non-verbal signs of anger include:
    A.   Pacing
    B.   Clenched fists
    C.   Reddened face or neck
    D.   Shouting
    E.   Rapid movements

23. Clients feel safer and more secure during a procedure if you:
    A.   Complete the procedure quickly
    B.   Explain why and how the procedure is done
    C.   Describe sensations or feelings they can expect
    D.   Explain who will do it

24. Which of the following behaviours can create barriers to effective communication?
    A.   Interrupting
    B.   Giving advice
    C.   Answering clients' questions
    D.   Minimizing problems
    E.   Using patronizing language
    F.   Failing to listen

25. Which of the following are steps in the four-step teaching method used when teaching a client a task?
    A.   Tell the client the steps in the task
    B.   Show the client how to do each task
    C.   Have the client try each step
    D.   Review what the client did wrong with each step

26. Which of the following are some of the other guidelines you can use when you are teaching tasks to clients?
    A.   Put the client at ease
    B.   Start with small, easy steps
    C.   Observe and listen
    D.   Make sure you set the pace
    E.   Allow for time to practise

27. Which of the following are the guidelines for dealing with an angry client?
    A. Ignore the client's feelings
    B. Treat the client with dignity and respect
    C. Tell the client what you are going to do and when
    D. Stay calm and professional
    E. Argue your point
    F. Listen and use silence
    G. Protect yourself from violent behaviours
    H. Report the client's behaviour to your supervisor

MULTIPLE CHOICE

Circle the correct answer.

28. Communication:
    A. Is a verbal account of client care and observations
    B. Is a written account of care and observations
    C. Uses the senses of sight, thought, and smell to collect information about a client
    D. Is the exchange of information

29. When you communicate assertively, you appear:
    A. Cold or angry
    B. Hesitant and timid
    C. Intimidated
    D. Confident and calm

30. You are teaching Mr. Simpson how to change his ostomy bag. You would:
    A. Explain all the steps necessary before starting the demonstration
    B. Teach him the hardest part first
    C. Use positive statements
    D. Set a time limit for him to complete the task

31. You are bathing Mrs. Fox when she suddenly starts to yell at you for not doing the bath correctly. Which of the following is an effective way to communicate with Mrs. Fox?
    A. Deny that you are doing it incorrectly
    B. Listen and remain calm
    C. Tell her you have been doing baths for many years and know what you are doing
    D. Stop the bath and leave the room

32. Asking closed questions:
    A. Invites a client to share thoughts or feelings
    B. Helps you to make sure you understand the client's message
    C. Focuses on specific information
    D. Helps you to find out about the client's needs

MATCHING

Match the description with the correct term.

33. _____ Restating someone's message in your own words

34. _____ Communicating positively and directly without offending others

35. _____ Questions that invite a client to share thoughts

36. _____ Paying close attention to a client's verbal and non-verbal communication

37. _____ Questions that focus on specific information

38. _____ Being attentive to a client's feelings

39. _____ Messages sent without words

40. _____ Limiting the conversation to a certain topic

41. _____ Gestures that send messages to others

42. _____ Spoken words

43. _____ Exchange of information between two people

A. Open-ended questions

B. Non-verbal communication

C. Paraphrasing

D. Verbal communication

E. Closed questions

F. Interpersonal communication

G. Empathetic listening

H. Body language

I. Active listening

J. Focusing

K. Assertiveness

CHAPTER 14

Body Structure and Function

TRUE OR FALSE

Circle T for true or F for false.

1. **T** F The skin is the body's first line of defence against disease.

2. **T** F The optic nerve is found in the ear.

3. **T** F The immune system is made up of red blood cells.

4. **T** F The tympanic membrane is found in the ear.

5. **T** F Fingernails and toenails are part of the integumentary system.

6. **T** F The peripheral nervous system is made up of the brain and spinal cord.

7. **T** F The parasympathetic nervous system is responsible for flight, fright, or fight.

8. **T** F Bones are dead.

9. **T** F A function of the muscular system is to provide the body with heat.

10. **T** F The function of the urinary system is to remove waste products from the blood.

11. **T** F The process of cell division is called mitosis.

12. **T** F The ball and socket joint allows movement in all directions.

13. **T** F The hinge joint allows turning from side to side.

14. **T** F The pivot joint allows movement in one direction.

15. **T** F The pathways that conduct messages to and from the brain are contained in the spinal cord.

16. **T** F The small bones in the middle ear are called the malleus, incus, and anvil.

17. **T**   **F**   The function of the lungs is to allow respiration.

18. **T**   **F**   Urine is made up of waste products filtered out of the liver.

19. **T**   **F**   The master gland of the endocrine system is the pituitary gland.

20. **T**   **F**   The major function of the thyroid gland is to regulate calcium.

21. **T**   **F**   Glucocorticoids regulate the metabolism of carbohydrates.

MULTIPLE RESPONSE

From the list below, choose all of the correct answers.

22. What are the basic structures of the cell?
    A.   Cell membrane
    B.   Nucleus
    C.   Pleura
    D.   Cytoplasm
    E.   Synovial fluid

23. Which of the following are the structures that make up the circulatory system?
    A.   Blood
    B.   Kidney
    C.   Heart
    D.   Vessels
    E.   Spinal cord

MULTIPLE CHOICE

Circle the correct answer.

24. What is the name of the body function that burns food for heat and energy?
    A.   Metabolism
    B.   Digestion
    C.   Peristalsis
    D.   Urination

25. The urinary system consists of:
    A.   2 kidneys, 2 ureters
    B.   2 kidneys, 1 bladder, ureters
    C.   Urethra and bladder
    D.   2 kidneys, 2 ureters, bladder, urethra

26. Smooth muscles may be found in the:
    A.   Arms and legs
    B.   Body track
    C.   Digestive tract
    D.   Head and neck

27. Each system of the body is composed of:
    A.   Cells, tissues, and bones
    B.   Tissues, organs, and muscles
    C.   Bones, muscles, and tissues
    D.   Cells, tissues, and organs

28. The middle layer of the skin is called the:
    A.   Epidermis
    B.   Dermis
    C.   Subcutaneous
    D.   Fat

29. What type of blood vessel carries blood away from the heart?
    A.   Artery
    B.   Vein
    C.   Vena cava
    D.   Capillary

30. The highest functions of the brain take place in the:
    A.   Cerebral cortex
    B.   Medulla
    C.   Brain stem
    D.   Spinal nerve

31. The endocrine glands secrete substances called:
    A.   Hormones
    B.   Mucus
    C.   Semen
    D.   Insulin

32. What is the major function of the thyroid gland?
   A. Regulates growth
   B. Prevents excessive loss of fluids
   C. Regulates metabolism
   D. Regulates calcium use by the body

33. Besides serving as the organ of hearing, the ear is involved with:
   A. Balance
   B. Regulating body movements
   C. Controlling involuntary muscles
   D. Smoothness of body movements

MATCHING

Match the following statements with the correct terms.

34. _____ Blood vessel that carries blood away from the heart

35. _____ Blood vessel that carries blood back to the heart

36. _____ Tiny blood vessel that allows food, oxygen, and other substances to pass to the cells

37. _____ Basic unit of body structure

38. _____ Group of cells with the same function

39. _____ Group of tissues with the same function

40. _____ Organs that work together to perform special functions

41. _____ Process of physically and chemically breaking down food so it can be absorbed for use by the cells of the body

42. _____ Muscle contractions in the digestive system that move food through the alimentary canal

43. _____ Burning of food by the cells to produce heat and energy

A. Artery
B. Capillary
C. Cell
D. Digestion
E. Metabolism
F. Organ
G. Peristalsis
H. System
I. Tissue
J. Vein

Match the four basic types of tissue with their functions.

44. _____ Epithelial tissue

45. _____ Connective tissue

46. _____ Muscle tissue

47. _____ Nerve tissue

A. Anchors, connects, and supports other body tissues
B. Relays information to and from the brain and throughout the body
C. Allows the body to move by stretching and contracting
D. Covers internal and external body surfaces

Match the bone with the correct description of what the bone does.

48. _____ Long bones   A. Allow skill and ease in movement

49. _____ Short bones   B. Protect the organs

50. _____ Flat bones   C. Bear the weight of the body

51. _____ Irregular bones   D. Allow various degrees of movement and flexibility

Match the following statements with one of the terms related to the digestive and urinary system.

52. _____ Structure that adds digestive juices to chyme   A. Bladder

53. _____ Semi-liquid food mixture formed in stomach   B. Chyme

54. _____ Portion of the gastrointestinal tract that absorbs food   C. Colon

55. _____ Portion of the gastrointestinal tract that absorbs water   D. Duodenum

56. _____ Produces digestive juices   E. Jejunum

57. _____ Produces bile   F. Kidney

58. _____ Basic working unit of the kidney   G. Liver

59. _____ Hollow muscular sac that stores urine   H. Meatus

60. _____ Structure that allows urine to pass from the bladder   I. Nephron

61. _____ Opening from the bladder at the end of the urethra   J. Pancreas

62. _____ Bean-shaped structure that produces urine   K. Urethra

63. _____ Moistens food particles in the mouth   L. Saliva

Match the correct pituitary hormone with the effect it has on the body.

64. _____ Growth hormone   A. Enables thyroid gland function

65. _____ Thyroid-stimulating hormone (TSH)   B. Prevents the kidneys from excreting excessive amounts of water

66. _____ Adrenocorticotropic hormone (ACTH)   C. Causes the uterine muscles to contract during childbirth

67. _____ Antidiuretic hormone (ADH)   D. Causes growth of muscles, bones, and other organs

68. _____ Oxytocin   E. Stimulates the adrenal gland

Match the action of the hormone with the correct hormone.

69. _____   Released by pancreas and regulates sugar in blood

70. _____   Sex hormone secreted by testes

71. _____   Sex hormone secreted by ovaries

72. _____   Regulates metabolism

73. _____   Regulates calcium levels in body

74. _____   Stimulates body to produce energy during emergencies

A.   Epinephrine

B.   Estrogen

C.   Insulin

D.   Parathyroid hormone

E.   Testosterone

F.   Thyroxine

Match the special cells or substances in the immune system to their function in protecting the body.

75. _____   Antibodies

76. _____   Antigens

77. _____   Phagocytes

78. _____   Lymphocytes

79. _____   B lymphocytes (B cells)

80. _____   T lymphocytes (T cells)

A.   Cause the body to produce antibodies

B.   Produce antibodies

C.   Cause the production of antibodies that circulate in the plasma

D.   Destroy invading cells or attract other cells that destroy invading cells

E.   Attack and destroy abnormal or unwanted substances

F.   Digest and destroy micro-organisms and other unwanted substances

Match the type of joint to each drawing

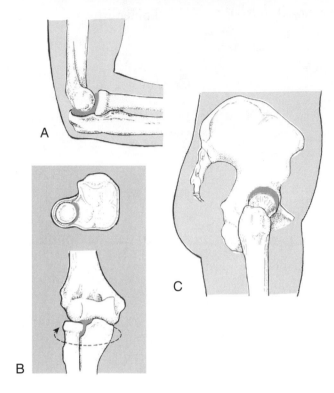

81. _____ Ball and socket

82. _____ Hinge joint

83. _____ Pivot joint

Match the parts of the brain to the areas indicated on the drawing

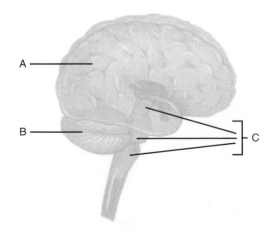

84. _____ Brain stem

85. _____ Cerebrum

86. _____ Cerebellum

Match the structure and function of the six main parts of the heart to the areas indicated on the drawing

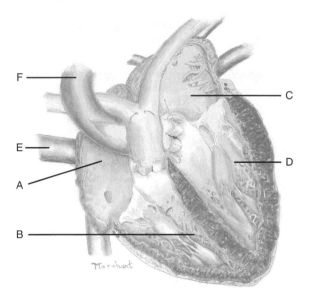

87. _____ Left atrium: Receives oxygenated blood from the lungs

88. _____ Left ventricle: Pumps oxygenated blood to all parts of the body

89. _____ Right atrium: Receives blood from body tissues

90. _____ Superior vena cava: Carries blood from the head and arms to the right atrium

91. _____ Aorta: A large artery that receives blood directly from the left ventricle and then branches into other arteries that carry the blood to all parts of the body

92. _____ Right ventricle: Pumps blood to the lungs for oxygen

Match the structures of the respiratory system to the areas indicated on the drawing

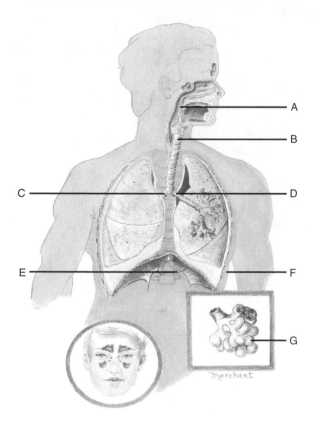

Match the structures of the digestive system to the areas indicated on the drawing

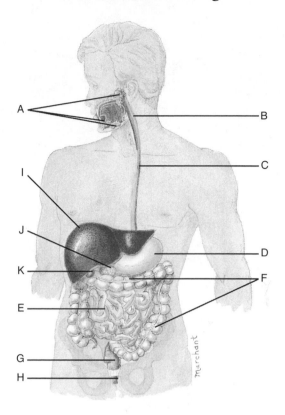

93. _____   Diaphragm

94. _____   Left main bronchus

95. _____   Pharynx

96. _____   Alveolus

97. _____   Trachea

98. _____   Right main bronchus

99. _____   Pleura

100. _____   Stomach

101. _____   Large intestine

102. _____   Small intestine

103. _____   Salivary glands

104. _____   Gall bladder

105. _____   Liver

106. _____   Esophagus

107. _____   Pancreas

108. _____   Pharynx (throat)

109. _____   Anus

110. _____   Rectum

Match the structures of the urinary system to the areas indicated on the drawing

Match the structures of the parts of the male reproductive system to the areas indicated on the drawing

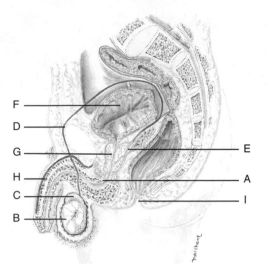

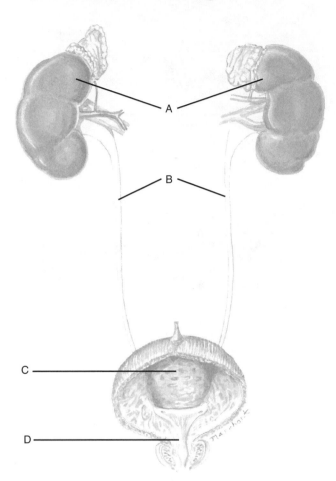

111. _____   Urinary bladder

112. _____   Urethra

113. _____   Kidneys

114. _____   Ureters

115. _____   Urinary bladder

116. _____   Anus

117. _____   Prostate gland

118. _____   Urethra

119. _____   Epididymis

120. _____   Penis

121. _____   Testis

122. _____   Vas deferens

123. _____   Seminal vesicle

Match the structures of the external female genitalia to the areas indicated on the drawing

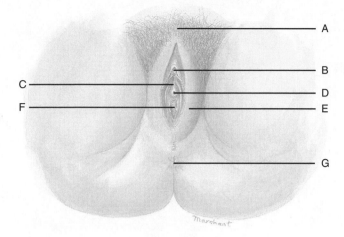

124. _____   Labia majora

125. _____   Labia minora

126. _____   Anus

127. _____   Mons pubis

128. _____   Vagina

129. _____   Urethra

130. _____   Clitoris

CHAPTER 15

Growth and Development

TRUE OR FALSE

Circle T for true or F for false.

1. **(T)** F   Three-month-old infants can raise their heads and shoulders when lying on their stomachs.

2. T   **(F)**   Toilet training is usually completed by the age of 1 ½ years.

3. **(T)** F   Three-year-olds are able to play with other children.

4. T   **(F)**   Young adulthood is the time when partners spend more time alone together.

5. **(T)** F   Adolescents begin to think about careers and what to do after high school graduation.

6. **(T)** F   The term *growth* refers to the physical changes that can be measured and that occur in a steady and organized manner.

7. **(T)** F   Development is a change in psychological and social functioning.

8. T   **(F)**   A *fetus* is a baby in the first 4 weeks after birth.

9. T   **(F)**   A 4-year-old child has a strong preference for the parent of the same sex.

10. **(T)** F   At 8 years of age, peer-group activities and opinions are important to the child.

11. **(T)** F   Puberty begins when reproductive organs begin to function.

12. T   **(F)**   During young adulthood, hobbies and pastimes can be pursued since more free time is available.

MULTIPLE RESPONSE

From the list below, choose all the correct answers.

13. Which of these are among the six basic principles of growth and development?
    A. Growth and development occur from the moment of birth until death.
    B. The process is simple to complex.
    C. Growth and development occur from head to foot and from the centre of the body outward.
    D. Growth and development occur in a sequence, order, and pattern; each stage lays the foundation for the next stage.
    E. Growth and development occur from the moment of fertilization until death.
    F. Growth and development occur at a set pace.
    G. Each stage of growth and development has its own characteristics and developmental tasks.

MULTIPLE CHOICE

Circle the correct answer.

14. The stage of infancy is the first:
    A. 4 weeks of life
    B. 3 months of life
    C. 6 months of life
    D. Year of life

15. Which reflexes does the infant need for feeding?
    A. The Moro and startle reflexes
    B. The rooting and sucking reflexes
    C. The grasping and Moro reflexes
    D. The rooting and grasping reflexes

16. At what age are solid foods usually given to an infant need for feeding?
    A. Fifth to seventh month
    B. Eighth month
    C. Ninth or tenth month
    D. Eleventh or twelfth month

17. Which of the following activities can a toddler do?
    A. Use a spoon and cup
    B. Ride a bike
    C. Help set the table
    D. Name parts of the body

18. During which stage do children begin playing with other children?
    A. Infancy
    B. The toddler years
    C. The preschool years
    D. Middle childhood

19. Reproductive organs begin to function and secondary sex characteristics appear during which stage?
    A. Late childhood
    B. Preadolescence
    C. Puberty
    D. Early adulthood

20. Middle adulthood is from about:
    A. 25 to 35 years
    B. 30 to 40 years
    C. 40 to 50 years
    D. 40 to 65 years

21. Middle adulthood is usually a time when:
    A. Families are started
    B. Physical energy and free time are gained
    C. Children are grown and leave home
    D. People need to prepare for death

22. What stage of growth and development includes the following developmental tasks: adjusting to physical changes; having grown children; developing leisure-time activities; and relating to aging parents?
A. Late adulthood
B. Young adulthood
C. Middle adulthood
D. Old adulthood

23. What stage of growth and development includes the following developmental tasks: increasing the ability to communicate with and understand others; performing self-care activities; learning the differences between the sexes and developing sexual modesty; learning right from wrong and good from bad; learning to play with others; and developing family relationships?
A. Puberty
B. Young adulthood
C. Preschool
D. Newborn

MATCHING

Match the correct age at which a child is expected to develop each of the following skills.

24. __G__ Speaks in short sentences
25. __H__ Usually protective of younger brothers and sisters
26. __I__ Learns to write in cursive script rather than print
27. __A__ Smiles and follows objects with the eyes
28. __F__ Can eat table food
29. __B__ Can hold a rattle
30. __E__ Reacts to the word "no"
31. __D__ Begins to bite and chew finger foods
32. __C__ Plays with the toes

A. 2 months
B. 3 months
C. 5 months
D. 6 months
E. 8 months
F. 1 year
G. 3 years
H. 5 years
I. 7 years

Match the behaviour or physical change with the correct age.

33. __H__ Do not like being teased or criticized and are sensitive about how others treat them

34. __C__ Temper tantrums and saying "no" are common

35. __J__ In girls, pelvis becomes broader, fat appears on hips and chest, and budding of breasts occurs

36. __A__ Movements are uncoordinated and lack purpose

37. __L__ Select partner and learn to live together; develop intimate relationships

38. __B__ May be able to stand when holding on to something

39. __D__ Bowel training usually is complete

40. __K__ Awkward movements occur because of rapid growth in height and weight

41. __E__ Recognize that male and female bodies are different

42. __I__ More permanent teeth appear; movements are faster and more graceful

43. __M__ Weight control becomes a problem as metabolism and physical activity slow down

44. __F__ May cheat to win, but they like rules and try to follow them

45. __G__ Baby teeth are lost, and replacement with permanent teeth begins

A. Birth–4 weeks

B. 8 months

C. 2 years

D. 2 ½ years

E. 3 years

F. 5 years

G. 6 years

H. 7 years

I. 8 years

J. 10–14 years

K. Adolescent

L. Young adulthood

M. Middle adulthood

Match the following statements with the correct reflex of an infant.

46. ___C___ Produced by touching the cheeks

47. ___B___ When cheek is touched, baby turns head in the direction of touch

48. ___A___ A loud noise causes infant to throw arms apart and extend legs

49. ___D___ When palm of hand is touched, baby closes fingers around object

A.   Moro (startle) reflex

B.   Rooting reflex

C.   Sucking reflex

D.   Grasping reflex

Match the developmental task with the correct age group.

50. ___F___ Accepting the changes in body and appearance

51. ___H___ Developing leisure-time activities

52. ___B___ Gaining control of bowel and bladder functions

53. ___D___ Becoming independent from parents and adults

54. ___A___ Learning to eat solid foods

55. ___E___ Developing a conscience and morals

56. ___C___ Learning to get along with peers

57. ___G___ Developing a satisfactory sex life

A.   Infancy (birth to 1 year)

B.   Toddler (1 to 3 years)

C.   Preschooler (3 to 6 years)

D.   Middle childhood (6 to 8 years)

E.   Late childhood (9 to 12 years)

F.   Adolescence (12 to 18 years)

G.   Young adulthood (18 to 40 years)

H.   Middle adulthood (40 to 65 years)

Match the developmental task with the correct age group.

58. __E__ Developing new friends and keeping friendships with peers

59. __B__ Using words to communicate with others

60. __G__ Learning to live with a partner

61. __D__ Developing a good feeling and attitude about self

62. __A__ Developing stable sleep and feeding patterns

63. __C__ Performing self-care activities

64. __F__ Accepting male or female role appropriate for one's age

A. Infancy (birth to 1 year)

B. Toddler (1 to 3 years)

C. Preschooler (3 to 6 years)

D. Middle childhood (6 to 8 years)

E. Late childhood (9 to 12 years)

F. Adolescence (12 to 18 years)

G. Young adulthood (18 to 40 years)

CHAPTER 16

Caring for the Young

TRUE OR FALSE

Circle T for true or F for false.

1. **T   F**   Do not tie pacifiers or other items around a baby's neck.

2. **T   F**   Position infants on their stomach in the crib.

3. **T   F**   It is not your duty to provide a stable, secure, or safe atmosphere for the family.

4. **T   F**   You should try to develop positive relationships with all family members.

5. **T   F**   You should punish the misbehaving child the way the parents would.

6. **T   F**   Bedtime rituals should be eliminated if the child is ill.

7. **T   F**   Sudden departure of a caregiver should be reported immediately.

8. **T   F**   Touching the child to provide comfort should depend on the child's culture.

MULTIPLE RESPONSE

From the list below, choose all of the correct answers.

9. Which of the statements below are true in preventing injuries in infants and children?
   A. Only use baby walkers outside.
   B. Keep the highchair away from stoves, tables, and counters.
   C. Secure the child into a highchair using the waist and crotch straps.
   D. Keep crib rails up and locked.
   E. Check children in cribs once a night.
   F. Make sure there are no toys or soft, fluffy items in the crib.
   G. Ensure the crib mattress is soft and bendable.
   H. Avoid using safety plugs in electrical outlets.
   I. Do not let electrical cords hang down from tables or counters.
   J. Do not let children wear necklaces, strings, cords, or other items around their necks.
   K. Hang items with strings, cords, or elastic only around cribs or playpens.
   L. Keep all poisonous substances in a high, locked area away from children.

M. Do not store harmful substances in food containers or juice bottles.

N. Keep childproof caps on harmful substances.

10. Ways to prevent children from drowning in or around the home include:
    A. Teaching children how to swim at a young age if they play near swimming pools unattended
    B. Keeping bathroom doors closed to prevent drowning in toilets or bathtubs
    C. Keeping diaper pails locked
    D. Keeping sinks, tubs, basins, and buckets empty when not in use

11. What safety measures can prevent burns in children?
    A. Do not drink cold liquids around children.
    B. Make sure children are not around hot utensils, irons, or dishes from the oven.
    C. Only heat a baby bottle in the microwave.
    D. Always shake the contents of a baby bottle thoroughly before giving it to the baby.
    E. Test the temperature of food and fluids before you give them to the baby.
    F. Always test bath water using your hand.
    G. Do not let a child touch faucet handles.
    H. Keep pot handles facing inward on the stove, away from a child's reach.
    I. Do not let children cook at the stove.
    J. Do not let children near curling irons or electric curlers.
    K. Do not let electric cords from irons, coffee pots, toasters, and so on hang down where a child can reach them.
    L. Do not let children play around ovens, fireplaces, or other heat sources.
    M. Supervise a child lighting firecrackers.
    N. Do not let a child play unsupervised outdoors if there are open firepits or burning leaves in the yard.

12. What measures can help to prevent poisoning in children?
    A. Keep all harmful substances in high, locked areas where children or confused adults cannot reach them.
    B. Discard old medications down the toilet.
    C. Store all harmful substances in their original containers.
    D. Never store harmful materials or liquids in food or juice containers.
    E. Never store harmful materials near foods.
    F. Never mix cleaning products, as mixing them could produce harmful fumes.
    G. Never call medications or vitamins "candy."
    H. Do not leave your purse or work bag sitting out where children can reach it, especially if it contains medications or harmful substances.
    I. Keep plants away from toddlers or infants.
    J. Do not let children play near walls with chipped paint. This paint may contain lead.
    K. Keep phone numbers for the Poison Control Centre, police, and ambulance handy near the phone.

MULTIPLE CHOICE

Circle the correct answer.

13. How can you prevent choking injuries?
    A. Use rolled towels to prop up bottles while baby is feeding.
    B. Never give infants and young children foods such as hot dogs, peanuts, or popcorn.
    C. Always use strings or cords to secure a child's hood and waistline.
    D. Position infants on their stomachs for sleep.

14. Children are vaccinated to _____ certain contagious infections.
    A. Prevent them from catching
    B. Cure them of
    C. Reduce the symptoms of
    D. Infect them with

15. Which of the following statements about vaccinating children is true?
    A. If vaccinations were to be discontinued, the rate of disease would go down.
    B. Children need to be vaccinated against viral meningitis.
    C. Vaccines can be given to infants only.
    D. Vaccinations prevent the spread of a certain variety of pathogens.

16. As a general rule, children should stay home from school or day care if:
    A. They drink normally but pick at their food
    B. They have a temperature of 37.5°C (99.5°F) and sleep soundly at night
    C. They have a temperature over 38°C (100.4°F), diarrhea, and vomiting
    D. They have been on antibiotics for 36 hours

17. Reye's syndrome is:
    A. A rare congenital condition caused by nuclear radiation
    B. A rare but often fatal illness linked to taking aspirin to treat influenza or chicken pox
    C. A condition caused by an allergy to acetaminophen (Tylenol)
    D. A common congenital condition caused by a mother drinking alcohol while pregnant

18. One of the five most common reasons children stay home from school or day care is that they:
    A. Have chicken pox
    B. Ate too many hot dogs at a birthday party
    C. Have test anxiety
    D. Have conjunctivitis

19. One of the main principles in supporting challenging children is to:
    A. Sternly punish bad behaviours
    B. Encourage and reinforce good behaviours
    C. Yell at them to let them know who is the boss
    D. Never give in to their demands

MATCHING

Match the safety measure used with the correct risk factor.

20. _____ Never store cleaning products in easy-to-reach areas.

21. _____ Measure the temperature of bath water.

22. _____ Keep one hand on a child lying on a table if you must look away.

23. _____ Do not prop up a baby bottle with a rolled-up towel or blanket.

A. Burns

B. Suffocation

C. Falls

D. Poisoning

Match the safety measure used with the correct risk factor.

24. _____   Teach children not to eat unknown foods, leaves, stems, seeds, berries, nuts, or bark.

25. _____   Never leave children unattended in a bathtub.

26. _____   Keep cords for drapes, blinds, and shades out of reach of children.

27. _____   Make sure there is nothing in the crib that the baby can stand on (like large stuffed toys or firm bumper pads).

A.   Burns

B.   Suffocation

C.   Falls

D.   Poisoning

CHAPTER 17

Caring for Older Adults

TRUE OR FALSE

Circle T if the statement promotes a client's sexuality and F if it does not.

1. **T**   **F**   Encourage the client to wear a hospital gown at all times.

2. **T**   **F**   Protect the client's right to privacy.

3. **T**   **F**   Encourage the client to get counselling if the client's sexual attitudes are different from yours.

4. **T**   **F**   Knock before you enter a room.

5. **T**   **F**   Allow older clients the right to be sexual.

6. **T**   **F**   Discourage single older clients from developing new relationships.

7. **T**   **F**   Allow couples in the long-term care facility to share the same room.

8. **T**   **F**   Discourage a woman from shaving her underarms and legs.

For the following statements, circle T for true or F for false.

9. **T**   **F**   Separation from children can cause loneliness in the older client.

10. **T**   **F**   Men usually live longer than women.

11. **T**   **F**   Clients who do not speak English have a greater risk of suffering from loneliness and isolation.

12. **T**   **F**   The skin of an older person is fragile and easily injured.

13. **T**   **F**   The older adult may have decreased mobility, thus decreasing the risk of falls.

14. **T**   **F**   Activity and diet can slow the loss of bone and muscle strength.

15. **T**   **F**   Decreased kidney function may cause the urine to be more concentrated.

16. **T** **F** Men may have difficulty urinating because of prostate gland enlargement.

17. **T** **F** The support worker can help the client at risk for urinary tract infections by providing extra fluids.

MULTIPLE RESPONSE

From the list below, choose all of the correct answers.

18. How can the support worker promote normal breathing in the older client?
  A. Do not allow heavy linens to cover the client's chest.
  B. Turn and reposition the client at least every 4 hours.
  C. Encourage deep breathing.
  D. If the client is on bed rest, keep the head of the bed flat.
  E. Encourage activity.

19. What are some ways in which an older adult may express closeness and intimacy without having intercourse?
  A. Holding hands
  B. Touching
  C. Caressing
  D. Embracing

MULTIPLE CHOICE

Circle the correct answer.

20. Which of these statements describes sexuality?
  A. It involves the whole personality and the body.
  B. It is not influenced by social, cultural, and spiritual factors.
  C. It is not present from birth.
  D. It is not done for pleasure or to produce children.

21. Which of these statements is true about sexuality and the older adult?
  A. After menopause, women are no longer interested in having sexual relations.
  B. A man cannot have an erection when he gets older.
  C. Sexual relationships are psychologically and physically important to the older adult.
  D. Orgasm may be less intense and longer in duration.

22. Which of the following physical changes is most likely to cause confusion or behavioural changes in an older client?
  A. Respiratory infections
  B. Lack of exercise
  C. Reduced blood flow to the brain
  D. Poor fluid intake

23. Why does an older client usually require a bath only twice a week?
  A. Less exercise is done, so frequent bathing is unnecessary.
  B. Fewer baths decrease the possibility of injury from falls in the tub.
  C. Skin becomes drier with aging and is easily damaged by frequent bathing.
  D. Muscles atrophy and strength is reduced.

24. Why should you avoid applying heat to the feet of an older client?
  A. The skin is dry and has fewer oil glands.
  B. More fold lines and wrinkles appear in the skin.
  C. The feet may become infected more easily.
  D. Decreased sensitivity to heat may increase the risk of burns.

25. Older adults often complain that food has no taste. This happens because:
    A. Memory is shorter in older adults.
    B. The number of taste buds decreases with age.
    C. The ability to feel heat and cold decreases.
    D. A progressive loss of brain cells occurs.

FILL IN THE BLANK

Indicate whether the examples given are:

A. *A benefit of working*
B. *A benefit of retirement*
C. *A negative aspect of retirement*

26. _____ Time to travel

27. _____ More leisure time

28. _____ Poor health and aging

29. _____ Increased medical bills with less income

30. _____ Personal fulfillment and usefulness

31. _____ Friendships formed with coworkers

32. _____ Reduced income forces lifestyle changes

33. _____ Time to do as you wish

34. _____ Meeting basic needs of love, belonging, and self-esteem

35. _____ Reward for a lifetime of work

Indicate whether each of the effects of aging listed are:

A. *Physical*
B. *Psychological*
C. *Social*

36. _____ Greying hair

37. _____ Preparing for one's own death

38. _____ Death of a partner

39. _____ Slower movements

40. _____ Retirement

MATCHING

Match the statement about physical changes in the older person with the body system affected.

41. _____   Decrease in bone strength   A.   Integumentary

42. _____   Change in sleeping patterns   B.   Musculo-skeletal

43. _____   Less blood flows through narrowed arteries   C.   Nervous

44. _____   Folds, lines, and wrinkles appear   D.   Cardiovascular

45. _____   Lung tissue becomes less elastic   E.   Respiratory

46. _____   Decreased appetite   F.   Digestive

47. _____   Urine becomes concentrated   G.   Urinary

Match the correct body system to the care measures described.

48. _____   Performing range-of-motion exercises   A.   Integumentary

49. _____   Providing a sweater and a lap blanket for a client who is cold   B.   Nervous

50. _____   Allowing the older client to rest or nap more during the day   C.   Musculo-skeletal

51. _____   Placing the client in a semi-Fowler's position   D.   Respiratory

CHAPTER 18

Common Diseases and Conditions

TRUE OR FALSE

Circle T for true or F for false.

1. **T** **F** People who have osteoarthritis experience joint stiffness with activity and range-of-motion exercises.

2. **T** **F** Rheumatoid arthritis affects only the large weight-bearing joints.

3. **T** **F** Rheumatoid arthritis in children can affect growth and development.

4. **T** **F** Arthroplasty is done to cure arthritis.

5. **T** **F** People can help to prevent osteoporosis by taking calcium and having a regular exercise program.

6. **T** **F** When turning and repositioning a client with osteoporosis, you should move him or her quickly to prevent fractures.

7. **T** **F** You must protect a client with osteoporosis from falls because he or she is at high risk for joint injuries.

8. **T** **F** An infant who has a fracture may be a victim of child abuse.

9. **T** **F** Phantom limb pains occur when a client has had an amputation.

10. **T** **F** A stroke occurs when brain cells get too much oxygen and too many nutrients.

11. **T** **F** All clients with Parkinson's disease will have impaired mental function but should be treated with dignity and respect.

12. **T** **F** Multiple sclerosis is a short-term, acute disease.

13. **T** **F** A client with chronic obstructive pulmonary disease (COPD) is at risk for respiratory infections.

14. **T** **F** Tuberculosis is spread by contact with infectious materials.

15. **T** **F** You cannot contract tuberculosis through contact with a client who has the disease.

16. T   F   Angina pectoris occurs when vessels narrow and the heart pumps with more force.

17. T   F   Activity will usually relieve angina pain in 3 to 15 minutes.

18. T   F   A common term for a myocardial infarction is *heart attack*.

19. T   F   The goal of cardiac rehabilitation after a myocardial infarction is to prevent another attack.

20. T   F   When a client has renal calculi, you should strain the urine.

21. T   F   When a client has persistent renal failure, only the renal system is affected.

22. T   F   If a client is vomiting, you need to follow Standard Practices.

23. T   F   A client who has human immunodeficiency virus (HIV) but has not developed acquired immune deficiency syndrome (AIDS) cannot infect others with the virus.

24. T   F   Elevated toilet seats are helpful to a client with osteoarthritis when the client has limited range of motion in the hips and knees.

25. T   F   Juvenile rheumatoid arthritis occurs in children.

26. T   F   Preventing deformities is one of the goals in treating rheumatoid arthritis.

27. T   F   When a client has osteoporosis, a fracture can occur because the bones are very brittle.

28. T   F   A client with Parkinson's disease does not need assistance with speech.

29. T   F   A client with emphysema can breathe more easily if he or she is allowed to sit upright and slightly forward.

30. T   F   Exercise and physical therapy can help a client with Parkinson's disease improve or maintain strength, posture, balance, and mobility.

31. T   F   Repeated asthma attacks can damage the respiratory system.

32. T   F   Tuberculosis bacteria is spread through contact.

33. T   F   When caring for a client with tuberculosis, you dispose of tissues by placing them in the garbage.

34. T   F   Blood pressure tends to rise with age, beginning at about age 55.

35. T   F   Hypertension is more common among Canadians of South Asian, Aboriginal, and African descent.

36. T   F   The risk of hypertension increases if excess weight is stored around the abdomen.

37. T   F   Good skin care and regular position changes can help to prevent skin breakdown.

38. T   F   With persistent renal failure, the nephrons of the kidneys are destroyed.

39. T   F   Clients with persistent renal failure have dialysis to remove wastes and excess water from the blood.

40. **T   F**   The most important way to prevent the spread of hepatitis is by practising Standard Practices.

41. **T   F**   AIDS reduces the client's ability to fight infections.

42. **T   F**   The use of condoms will help prevent the spread of sexually transmitted infections (STIs).

MULTIPLE RESPONSE

From the list below, choose all of the correct answers.

43. Which of the following are early warning signs of cancer?
    A.   A cough that goes on for more than two days
    B.   Blood in the stool
    C.   Indigestion that continues more than an hour
    D.   Unexplained aches and pains that go on for more than two weeks
    E.   Difficulty urinating or blood in the urine
    F.   Bleeding after a cut
    G.   Any lump or mass
    H.   A sore that does not heal
    I.   A new growth on the skin
    J.   Patches of skin that bleed, itch, or are red

44. What side effects of radiation therapy cause clients with cancer to have special care needs?
    A.   Discomfort
    B.   Nausea and vomiting
    C.   Increased appetite
    D.   Fatigue
    E.   Diarrhea
    F.   Skin breakdown

45. A child falls and has signs and symptoms of a fracture. These would include which of the following?
    A.   Limb looks bent or out of position
    B.   Pain
    C.   Swelling
    D.   Unlimited movement of limb
    E.   Bruising and colour changes in the skin at the fracture site
    F.   Bleeding (internal or external)

46. What treatments are used to relieve pain and stiffness in a client with osteoarthritis?
    A.   Physicians may order aspirin for pain.
    B.   Heat or cold applications may be ordered.
    C.   Obese clients may be advised to gain weight.
    D.   A low-fat, low-calorie diet may be ordered.
    E.   A cane or walker may be used for support.

47. Which of the following are rules you should follow when caring for a client with a cast?
    A.   Make sure to cover the cast with blankets, plastic, or other material.
    B.   Turn the client as directed by the care plan.
    C.   Place a wet cast on a hard surface.
    D.   Support a wet cast with your palms when turning and positioning the client.
    E.   Protect the client from rough cast edges.
    F.   Keep a plaster cast dry.
    G.   Do not allow the client to insert anything into the cast.
    H.   Elevate a casted arm or leg on pillows.
    I.   Have enough help when turning and repositioning the client.
    J.   Position the client as directed by your supervisor and the care plan.

48. When you care for a client with a hip fracture, what measures are important for you to follow?
    A. Meet basic needs if the client is confined to bed, and prevent complications of bed rest.
    B. Transfer, turn, and reposition the person as directed.
    C. Keep the operated leg adducted at all times.
    D. Encourage external rotation of the hip.
    E. Provide range-of-motion exercises as directed.
    F. Provide a straight-backed chair with armrests.
    G. Place the chair on the affected side.
    H. Do not let the client stand on the affected leg unless allowed by the physician.
    I. Support and elevate the leg as directed when the client is in a chair.
    J. Apply elastic stockings as directed.
    K. Remind the client that it is okay to cross the legs while seated.

49. If you are caring for a client who has had a stroke, you might observe effects such as:
    A. Hemiplegia
    B. Weakness on both sides of the body
    C. Loss of face control
    D. Changing emotions
    E. Difficulty swallowing
    F. Dimmed vision or loss of vision
    G. Improved ability to speak or understand others
    H. Changes in sight, touch, movement, and thought
    I. Improved memory
    J. Urinary frequency, urgency, or incontinence

50. What measures would be helpful to use when you care for a client who has had a stroke?
    A. Complete all activities of daily living for the client.
    B. Encourage the client to do as little as possible.
    C. Meet basic needs if the client is confined to bed; prevent complications of bed rest.
    D. Assist with bladder or bowel training programs.
    E. Assist with range-of-motion exercises.
    F. Provide emotional support and encouragement.
    G. Report any changes in the person's mood or behaviour.

51. Infants and children may suffer brain damage from acquired brain injuries caused by:
    A. Conditions during birth
    B. Being shaken
    C. Childhood diseases
    D. Accidents

52. How can you help the client with pneumonia to breathe more easily and be more comfortable?
    A. Limit fluid intake.
    B. Position the client in Fowler's or semi-Fowler's position.
    C. Assist with oxygen therapy, as needed.

53. What damage can hypertension do to other body organs?
    A. The heart may enlarge.
    B. Blood vessels in the brain may burst and cause a stroke.
    C. Blood vessels in the eyes may be damaged.
    D. Blood vessels in the kidneys (and other organs) may be damaged.

54. Which risk factors of coronary artery disease can be changed by the client through lifestyle changes?
    A. Lack of exercise
    B. Excessive weight
    C. Smoking
    D. Excessive alcohol
    E. Stress
    F. Genetic link

55. What signs and symptoms would tell you a client is experiencing angina pectoris?
    A. Pain on the right side that may travel (radiate) to the jaw, neck, shoulders, back, and arms
    B. Shortness of breath
    C. Nausea
    D. Dry skin
    E. Dizziness or light-headedness
    F. Fatigue
    G. Palpitations

56. If a client is having a myocardial infarction, the signs and symptoms may include:
    A. Sudden, severe chest pain, usually on the right side
    B. Pain described as crushing, stabbing, or squeezing
    C. Pain that radiates to the neck and jaw, and down the arm or to the sides
    D. Pain that is more severe and lasts longer than angina
    E. Pain that is relieved by rest and nitroglycerin
    F. Indigestion
    G. Shortness of breath
    H. Nausea or vomiting
    I. Dizziness
    J. Perspiration
    K. Cyanosis
    L. Cold and clammy skin
    M. Low blood pressure
    N. Weak and irregular pulse

57. How is pain from angina relieved or avoided?
    A. Strenuous physical exertion
    B. Resting when the pain begins
    C. Avoiding stress
    D. Avoiding other triggers (extreme cold or heat, heavy meals, alcohol, smoking)
    E. Taking nitroglycerin
    F. Bypass surgery

58. When you are caring for a client with acute renal failure, the care plan is likely to include:
    A. Measure and record urine output every 6 hours
    B. Measure and record intake and output
    C. Increase fluid intake
    D. Weigh the client daily using a different scale
    E. Provide frequent oral hygiene
    F. Meet basic needs if the client is confined to bed; prevent complications of bed rest
    G. Prevent infections

59. What are the signs and symptoms of hepatitis?
    A. Nausea, vomiting, and abdominal pain
    B. Light-coloured urine
    C. Jaundice
    D. Dark-coloured stools
    E. Muscle pain
    F. Increased energy
    G. Irritability
    H. Itching
    I. Diarrhea
    J. General aching in the joints, accompanied by redness and swelling

60. Some complications of diabetes mellitus include:
    A. Blindness
    B. Kidney disease
    C. Nerve damage
    D. Sexual dysfunction
    E. Circulatory disorders
    F. Stroke and heart attack
    G. Improved wound healing

61. AIDS is spread by:
    A. Protected intercourse with an HIV-infected person
    B. Needle-sharing among IV drug users
    C. HIV-infected mothers to their babies at birth or during breastfeeding
    D. When infected body fluids (not including saliva, tears, urine, or sweat) come into direct contact with broken skin
    E. Needle stick injuries
    F. Casual contact such as hugging

62. What signs and symptoms may occur with both hypoglycemia and hyperglycemia?
    A. Hunger
    B. Vision changes
    C. Headache
    D. Slow pulse
    E. High blood pressure
    F. Confusion
    G. Convulsions
    H. Loss of consciousness

MULTIPLE CHOICE

Circle the correct answer.

63. If a client with rheumatoid arthritis tells you she has wrist pain, you would be correct to expect the pain to be:
    A. In the dominant hand
    B. In the non-dominant hand
    C. In both wrists
    D. None of the above

64. Which of the following is not a cause of osteoporosis?
    A. Lack of estrogen
    B. Regular exercise
    C. Lack of dietary calcium
    D. Bed rest and immobility

65. When caring for a client who had a hip replacement 5 weeks ago, which of these activities would not be allowed?
    A. Abduction of the affected leg
    B. Using an abductor splint or pillow between the legs when in bed
    C. Crossing the legs when sitting
    D. Using a shower chair for bathing

66. Gangrene can occur because of:
    A. Joint immobility and inflammation
    B. Infection, injuries, and decreased circulation
    C. Poor body alignment and positioning
    D. Porous, brittle bones

67. A transient ischemic attack (TIA):
    A. Is another name for a stroke
    B. Occurs when blood supply to the brain is disrupted for a short period
    C. Occurs when blood pressure is elevated
    D. Occurs when there is high sugar in the blood

68. The goal of rehabilitation in a client with a spinal cord injury is:
    A. To return to all normal activities
    B. To learn to function at the client's highest level
    C. To regain the use of the arms and legs
    D. To prevent further injury

69. You are caring for a client who has angina, and you find a bottle of tablets marked "Nitroglycerine" at the bedside. You should:
    A. Place them in a locked cabinet
    B. Tell the nurse
    C. Give them to the family to take home
    D. Make sure they remain where the client put them

70. Which of these measures would not be included in the treatment of a client with persistent heart failure?
    A. A diet high in salt
    B. Oxygen
    C. Drugs to strengthen the heart
    D. A semi-Fowler's or Fowler's position for easier breathing

71. Childhood communicable diseases are most commonly transmitted by:
    A. Airborne spread of or direct contact with respiratory secretions
    B. Direct contact with feces
    C. Direct contact with skin lesions
    D. Contact with a carrier

72. Which disease do the following signs and symptoms describe?
    Unusual mass or swelling, unexplained paleness or loss of energy, sudden tendency to bruise, persistent localized pain, or frequent headaches, especially with vomiting
    A. Stroke
    B. Emphysema
    C. Cancer
    D. Parkinson's disease

73. Which disease do the following signs and symptoms describe?
    Blurred or double vision, numbness and tingling, muscle weakness, difficulty speaking, dizziness, poor coordination, bladder problems
    A. Stroke
    B. Parkinson's disease
    C. Multiple sclerosis
    D. Emphysema

74. Which disease do the following signs and symptoms describe?
    Sudden weakness or numbness on one side of the body, impaired vision or loss of vision, loss of speech or trouble talking, loss of control of facial muscles, unexplained dizziness
    A. Stroke
    B. Parkinson's disease
    C. Multiple sclerosis
    D. Emphysema

75. Which disease do the following signs and symptoms describe?
    Enlarged alveoli, loss of elasticity in the walls of the alveoli. Air remaining trapped in the alveoli during expiration, shortness of breath and "smoker's cough," barrel chest
    A. Stroke
    B. Parkinson's disease
    C. Multiple sclerosis
    D. Emphysema

76. Which disease do the following signs and symptoms describe?
    Mask-like facial expression, tremors, pill-rolling movements of the fingers, shuffling gait, impaired balance, stooped posture, stiff muscles, slurred or monotone speech, drooling
    A. Cancer
    B. Parkinson's disease
    C. Multiple sclerosis
    D. Emphysema

77. Which area of the body would be paralyzed if the client had a cervical spine injury?
    A. From the neck down
    B. One side of the body
    C. From the chest down
    D. From the waist down

78. Spinal cord injuries at the thoracic level (chest area) or lower may cause:
    A. Quadriplegia
    B. Paralysis on one side of the body
    C. Paraplegia
    D. Paralysis of one limb

FILL IN THE BLANK

Indicate whether the symptom or physical effects listed relate to:

A. **Chronic bronchitis**
B. **Emphysema**

79. _____ Person develops barrel chest

80. _____ Mucus and inflamed breathing passages obstruct airflow

81. _____ Walls of alveoli are less elastic

Indicate whether the symptoms listed relate to:

A. **Hypoglycemia**
B. **Hyperglycemia**

82. _____ Trembling

83. _____ Nausea and vomiting

84. _____ Cold, clammy skin

85. _____ Flushed face

86. _____ Tiredness and fatigue

87. _____ Dizziness

88. _____ Dry skin

89. _____ Sweating

90. _____ Slow, laboured breathing

MATCHING

Match the three types of diabetes mellitus with the age or situation when each type usually occurs.

91. _____ Type 1 diabetes

92. _____ Type 2 diabetes

93. _____ Gestational diabetes

A. Develops during pregnancy

B. Occurs most often in children and young adults

C. Usually develops in adulthood

CHAPTER 19

Safety

TRUE OR FALSE

Circle T for true or F for false.

1. T F An electrical plug not being grounded may cause a fire.

2. T F Visitors need to be reminded not to smoke in a room with supplemental oxygen, even if the facility has a "No Smoking" policy.

3. T F To prevent sparks, you must turn off electrical equipment before unplugging it.

4. T F You should attempt to put out a fire before sounding a fire alarm.

5. T F All fire extinguishers are effective for any fire.

6. T F Disinfectants and cleaning solutions are hazardous substances.

7. T F Warnings, words, pictures, and symbols on hazardous substances may be removed after opening the container.

8. T F Check the material safety data sheet (MSDS) after cleaning up a leak or spill or disposing of a hazardous substance.

9. T F When using restraints, the most restrictive device is used.

10. T F Apply a restraint only after receiving instructions about its proper use.

11. T F Always follow manufacturers' instructions when using restraints.

12. T F Sheets, towels, or other items can be used to position and stabilize a client on the toilet.

MULTIPLE RESPONSE

From the list below, choose all of the correct answers.

13. What physical changes in some older adults place them at risk for accidents?
    A. Stiff joints and weakened muscle groups
    B. Improved balance and coordination
    C. Increased sensitivity to heat, smell, taste, and touch
    D. Diminished vision and hearing
    E. Memory problems

14. Why should you avoid calling a client by name as a method of identifying the client?
    A. Some clients may be confused and unaware of their name.
    B. Some clients who are disoriented may answer to any name.
    C. Some clients with hearing difficulties may not hear you correctly.

15. The support worker can prevent falls when giving care by:
    A. Taping cords and wires near the wall and away from the path for walking
    B. Using high-gloss floor wax to prevent tripping
    C. Cleaning up water and other spills immediately
    D. Keeping lights on low dimmers to decrease glare
    E. Reporting frayed, torn, or bumpy rugs and carpets
    F. Rearranging the client's furniture to a better arrangement
    G. Using non-slip rubber bath mats or non-slip strips in bathtubs and showers
    H. Making sure that the client's footwear and clothing fit properly
    I. Ensuring the client's shoes and slippers are non-skid

16. Injury prevention measures include:
    A. Encouraging the client to wear reading glasses when up and about
    B. Ensuring crutches, canes, and walkers have non-skid tips
    C. Checking the client carefully and often, especially a client with risk factors
    D. Using pillows, wedge pads, or seats to position the client as the care plan directs
    E. Keeping wheelchair wheels unlocked when stationary

17. Under the occupational health and safety (OH&S) legislation, what must your employer do to ensure your safety?
    A. Have written safety policies.
    B. Train and educate employees about these safety policies.
    C. Create a health and safety committee to identify workplace hazards and investigate accidents.
    D. Respond to reports of workplace hazards.
    E. Warn employees about safety hazards and correcting these hazards whenever possible.
    F. Make sure that all necessary equipment is available and in good working order.

18. What are the employee's responsibilities as outlined in the OH&S legislation?
    A. Following all safety policies and procedures
    B. Using all recommended protective equipment and clothing
    C. Deciding which concerns should be addressed to the supervisor or the health and safety committee
    D. Completing an incident report after an accident

19. Safety measures aimed at preventing burns include:
    A. Telling clients about the dangers of wearing tight-fitting clothing while cooking
    B. Keeping clients who smoke a designated distance away from the doors of the facility
    C. Following safety guidelines and the care plan when applying heat and cold
    D. Testing the temperature of food by dipping a clean spoon into the food and touching the inner aspect of your lower arm with it

E. Testing the water in the tub, shower, or basin with your hand before bathing an adult or helping an adult bathe

F. Checking for "hot spots" in water, and mix the water well by moving your hand back and forth in it

G. Relying on the client to check the temperature of the bathwater before bathing

H. Allowing the client to eat or drink food that is only warm and not hot

20. Incident reports are used by employers and health and safety committees to:
   A. Identify recurring problems
   B. Determine who is following health and safety policies
   C. Revise safety policies as needed
   D. Justify cost-saving measures

21. What safety information should the support worker know and use when handling hazardous substances?
   A. How to safely handle the product
   B. The cost of the product
   C. How to safely use the product
   D. How to safely freeze the product
   E. First aid measures required in case of an accident or emergency
   F. Instructions for disposing of the product

22. Call bells:
   A. Can be ignored if the client is known to call needlessly
   B. Should always be placed within the client's reach on their strong or dominant side
   C. Enable the client to call for assistance
   D. Can be removed from a client's bedside if the staff are frequently alerted

23. What information about hazardous materials can be found on the Workplace Hazardous Materials Information System (WHMIS) label?
   A. Risk phrases that describe the health hazard
   B. Supplier information
   C. Hazard symbol
   D. Cost of the product
   E. Precautionary statements that describe safety measures to take when using the product
   F. First aid measures in case of accident or emergency
   G. Reference to the material safety data sheet (MSDS)

24. Restraints may be used only:
   A. When absolutely necessary
   B. When the client is in imminent danger of harming others
   C. When a client is refusing to eat
   D. When a client actively threatens to harm himself
   E. As a last resort and after less-restrictive measures have failed

25. What are some client behaviours that would justify the use of restraints?
   A. A client tries to pull out an IV and feeding tube, and without these tubes, the client could die.
   B. A client is found by another client masturbating by himself in the dining room.
   C. A client with severe mental illness tries to strangle a staff member.
   D. A child tries to rip out her stitches, thus risking serious infection.
   E. A client is refusing to eat.

26. What alternatives to restraints can be used by a support worker when giving care?
    A. Use diversions, such as TV or music, to calm and distract the client
    B. Avoid following routines and habits since they obviously do not work
    C. Provide attention and companionship
    D. Turn up the volume of the TV or radio so the client will hear it
    E. Avoid explaining procedures and care measures to reduce confusion
    F. Closely supervise the client
    G. Allow the client to wander in a safe area
    H. Promote uninterrupted sleep
    I. Meet food, fluid, and elimination needs promptly
    J. If ordered, help the client use padded hip protectors, pillows, wedge cushions, and posture and positioning aids
    K. Follow safety precautions to prevent falls; if ordered, use floor cushions and roll guards
    L. Take away call bells, as they are a safety hazard

27. How can you meet a restrained client's psychological needs?
    A. Treat the person with kindness, caring, respect, and dignity
    B. Toilet the client every 6 hours
    C. Visit the person often
    D. Offer repeated explanations and reassurance
    E. Be a good listener

28. What information should be reported to the nurse when you are caring for a restrained client?
    A. The type of restraint applied
    B. The reason for the restraint
    C. Safety measures taken, as listed in the care plan, such as if bed rails are padded or raised
    D. The time the restraint was applied
    E. The time the restraint was removed

F. The care given when the restraint was removed
G. Skin colour and condition
H. The pulse felt in the restrained part
I. Complaints of a tight restraint, difficulty breathing, and pain, numbness, or tingling in the restrained part

MULTIPLE CHOICE

Circle the response that correctly completes the sentence.

29. A chemical restraint is a _____ used to control behaviour or movement.
    A. Belt
    B. Jacket
    C. Food
    D. Medication

30. If the support worker applies a restraint unnecessarily, he or she could face _____ charges.
    A. Assault
    B. False imprisonment
    C. Restraint
    D. False restraint

31. The client or substitute decision maker must give _____ for the use of restraints.
    A. Complete consent
    B. Informed consent
    C. Written permission
    D. Verbal permission

32. When a client is restrained, the support worker must check the client at least every _____.
    A. 5 minutes
    B. 15 minutes
    C. Hour
    D. 2 hours

33. The support worker must meet the restrained client's needs for _____, _____, _____, and _____.
    A. Fluid, clothing, shelter, elimination
    B. Food, fluid, shelter, entertainment
    C. Nutrition, clothing, comfort, entertainment
    D. Food, fluid, comfort, elimination

34. Several staff members may be needed to apply restraints to prevent a combative or agitated client from _____ themselves or the worker.
    A. Injuring
    B. Agitating
    C. Angering
    D. Upsetting

35. Several staff members apply restraints together in order to apply the restraint in a _____ manner.
    A. Safer
    B. Faster
    C. Safer and faster
    D. Correct and faster

36. Confusion may increase when a client is restrained because the client cannot _____ what is happening.
    A. See
    B. Hear
    C. Understand
    D. Help

37. When applying restraints, the client should be positioned in good body alignment and any bony areas and skin should be _____ to prevent _____ and injury.
    A. Covered, pressure
    B. Padded, pressure
    C. Covered, scratches
    D. Padded, scratches

38. Restraints that are too big or loose can increase the risk of _____.
    A. Cuts
    B. Bruises
    C. Strangulation
    D. Suffocation

39. When a client's clothing is on fire, you should _____ the client and cover him or her with a _____ or coat to smother the flames.
    A. Roll, blanket
    B. Hug, curtain
    C. Hug, blanket
    D. Roll, curtain

40. What are two safety problems with the plug shown in the figure?
    A. The cord is too big, and the plug is not grounded.
    B. The cord is frayed, and the plug is not grounded.
    C. The cord is too short, and the plug is the wrong shape.
    D. The cord is frayed, and the plug is the wrong shape.

MULTIPLE CHOICE

Circle the correct answer.

41. It is important to exercise personal safety measures at all times to avoid injury. If visiting a client in the home, one safety precaution would be to:
    A. Position yourself in the corner of the room
    B. Remove shoes or boots and throw them at the client
    C. Try to reason with the client or family member who is abusive or making sexual demands
    D. Be cautious in hallways, elevators, and stairwells

42. Which is a good personal safety measure to take when driving to and from work?
    A. Always use a seat belt
    B. Never park near people. Choose remote, empty areas
    C. Do not take your keys out until you are at your car
    D. Never carry cash with you at any time

43. If someone tries to force you into a vehicle, you should:
    A. Cry softly
    B. Push your thumbs into the attacker's eyes
    C. Avoid resisting and go into the vehicle
    D. Crouch in a fetal position

44. Where will you find information about a client's special safety needs?
    A. MSDS
    B. Client's care plan
    C. Kardex
    D. Medical record

45. Accident risk factors include:
    A. Natural disasters
    B. Impaired vision and hearing
    C. Suffocation
    D. Sleeping

46. Which of the following sets of factors puts a client at increased risk for falls?
    A. Confusion, disorientation, and memory problems
    B. Increased joint mobility and muscle strength
    C. Visual impairment, strange surroundings, and improved reaction time
    D. Regular exercise and diet habits, proper use of medications

47. Which of the following statements about the use of restraints is correct?
    A. Unnecessary restraint is false imprisonment.
    B. Clients who are confused usually become calmer after being restrained.
    C. Using restraints for as little time as possible improves quality of life.
    D. The least restrictive method must be used.

48. The restraint used is determined by the:
    A. Doctor's order
    B. Client's care plan
    C. Client's legal representative
    D. All of the above

49. Which of the following can result from restraint use?
    A. Cancer, urinary incontinence
    B. Hunger, humility, hypertension
    C. Increased sense of well-being and self-esteem
    D. Depression, embarrassment, humiliation, mistrust

50. Which of these statements is correct regarding restraints?
    A. Certain drugs may be a form of restraint.
    B. Restraints may be used for staff convenience.
    C. Restraints are never used to protect a client from harming himself or herself or others.
    D. The staff determines who should be restrained.

51. To identify a client:
    A. Call the client by his or her name
    B. Use the MSDS
    C. Use the client's ID bracelet
    D. Use the client's bed label

52. In a facility, falls are most likely to occur:
    A. During shift changes
    B. During meal times
    C. When visitors are present
    D. While care is being given

53. Which factor increases a client's risk for falling?
    A. Awareness of surroundings
    B. A history of falls
    C. Well-fitting footwear
    D. Muscle coordination

54. A client who has balance problems is:
    A. At risk for memory problems
    B. Suffering from impaired hearing
    C. At risk for falling
    D. Taking medication

55. Which of the following can help to prevent falls?
    A. Spills on the floor
    B. Scatter rugs
    C. Night lights
    D. Clutter

56. A person has a chair alarm. Which is true?
    A. It serves the same purpose as a night light.
    B. You need to respond immediately to the alarm.
    C. Alarms are used only at night.
    D. Alarms reduce the need to watch the client.

57. Bed rails are padded to:
    A. Prevent the person from getting caught between the rails and the mattress
    B. Provide privacy for the person
    C. Prevent the person from climbing out of bed
    D. Decrease agitation

58. What should you do if you find that a smoke detector does not work in a home where you are giving care?
    A. Replace the battery.
    B. Call the fire department.
    C. Notify the nurse and the family.
    D. This is not your responsibility; do not get involved.

59. If a fire occurs, which of these steps should be done first?
    A. Use a fire extinguisher to put out the fire.
    B. Close all doors and windows.
    C. Sound the nearest fire alarm.
    D. Move people who are in danger to a safe place.

60. Suffocation can occur because:
    A. A person chokes on a piece of food
    B. A person is given a tub bath
    C. Restraints are applied correctly
    D. Dentures fit properly

61. When an accident or error occurs, it is correct to:
    A. Report the accident or error immediately to your supervisor
    B. Report the incident only if a client is injured
    C. Call the family immediately
    D. Call the doctor or ambulance

62. If your car breaks down, a good safety practice would be to:
    A. Stay in the car and call police if you have a cellular phone
    B. Ask for a ride to a police station if someone stops to help
    C. Walk to the nearest place where you can get help
    D. Get out of the car and try to flag down a ride for help

63. If you feel uncomfortable or threatened in a home setting, you should first:
A. Speak to the person who is threatening you
B. Go to a safe place immediately and call your supervisor
C. Resign from your job
D. Call a coworker to come to the home to assist you

64. Which of the following would be a threat to your safety in home care?
A. Denial of meal breaks, drinking water, or bathroom use
B. Inadequate heat or ventilation
C. Being subject to name calling or obscene language
D. All of the above

MATCHING

Match the description or example with the correct restraint.

65. _____ A drug is given that is not required to treat the client's medical symptoms.

66. _____ An attached tray keeps the client from getting up.

67. _____ Hands are covered to prevent the client from removing the dressing.

A. Chemical restraint

B. Mitt restraint

C. Geriatric chair

Match the safety measure used with the correct risk factor.

68. _____ Measure the temperature of bath water.

69. _____ Keep the client's room free of clutter.

70. _____ Open doors and windows if you notice gas odours.

71. _____ Store cleaners, medicines, and hazardous substances in the original containers.

A. Burns

B. Suffocation

C. Falls

D. Poisoning

Match the safety measure used with the correct risk factor.

72. _____ Do not allow smoking in bed.

73. _____ Do not prop up a baby bottle with a rolled-up towel or blanket.

74. _____ Use non-slip strips on the floor next to the bed and in the bathroom.

A. Burns

B. Suffocation

C. Falls

Match the accident risk factor with the possible outcome or injury.

75. _____ Can harm herself or others because she cannot understand what is happening

76. _____ May take wrong medication or dosage or poison himself because cannot read labels

77. _____ Having problems smelling smoke or gas so is unaware of fire

78. _____ Cannot hear fire alarms or sirens, so cannot move to safety

79. _____ Has not learned the difference between safety and danger so is unaware of hazardous situation

80. _____ May be aware of danger but is unable to move to safety

A. Impaired awareness of surroundings

B. Impaired vision

C. Impaired hearing

D. Altered sense of smell or touch

E. Paralysis

F. Developmental stage or age

Match the accident risk factor with the possible outcome or injury.

81. _____ Injury resulting from being unaware that certain people, places, or things may be safety hazards

82. _____ Movements slower and less steady; balance affected

83. _____ Can trip on toys, rugs, furniture, electrical cords

84. _____ Easily burned because of problems sensing heat and cold

85. _____ Cannot hear explanation or instructions so may take wrong medication or dosage

86. _____ May develop pressure sores from lack of movement

87. _____ Unaware that mixing these without proper guidance can cause illness or death

A. Impaired awareness of surroundings

B. Impaired vision

C. Impaired hearing

D. Altered sense of touch

E. Paralysis

F. Medications

G. Developmental stage or age

CHAPTER 20

Preventing Infection

TRUE OR FALSE

Circle T for true or F for false.

1. T   F   Microbes get nourishment from the reservoir.

2. T   F   Microbes are destroyed by a warm, dark environment.

3. T   F   Items can be sterilized in the home with boiling water.

4. T   F   If you must transport a client who has an infection that requires droplet or airborne precautions out of his or her room, the client must wear a disposable gown.

5. T   F   When you remove gloves, the inside is considered clean.

6. T   F   If a sterile item touches a clean item, the sterile item is contaminated.

7. T   F   If a clean item touches a sterile item, the clean item is contaminated.

8. T   F   If a sterile item is above your waist, it is contaminated.

9. T   F   Microbes exist in six different forms.

10. T   F   Animals are common reservoirs for microbes.

11. T   F   The environment must be warm and bright for microbes to survive.

12. T   F   Hands should be held up throughout the handwashing procedure.

13. T   F   Paper towels are used to turn off hand-operated water faucets to avoid contaminating the hands.

14. T   F   Mr. Fox has an infection caused by a wound on his leg. This infection can exit Mr. Fox's body through his wound.

15. T   F   Pathogens from Mr. Fox's infection cannot enter another person's body through a portal of entry.

16. T   F   Portals of entry can include mucous membranes.

17. T   F   The easiest and most important way to prevent the spread of infection is by eating well and staying fit.

18. T   F   A gown is contaminated when wet and should be removed.

19. T   F   Nosocomial or health care–associated infections (HAI) are acquired after a person's release from a health care facility.

20. T   F   The respiratory tract is one of the most common sites for nosocomial infections.

21. T   F   When cleaning equipment, the support worker should rinse the item in cold water first.

22. T   F   Chemical disinfectants are used to clean reusable items.

23. T   F   An effective and cheap disinfectant for home use may be made by mixing 1 cup of bleach with 3 cups of water.

24. T   F   After preparing the effective and cheap disinfectant solution from question #23, it should be labelled "toxic cleaner."

25. T   F   A simple way to sterilize items in the home is to pour boiling water over them.

26. T   F   If an item is sitting on the floor, it is considered to be contaminated.

27. T   F   When you are finished using a sharp object (such as a razor), after giving care, you should place it in the garbage.

28. T   F   After being worn, the outside part of a mask is considered to be contaminated.

29. T   F   Gloves should be changed between tasks (procedures) on the same client.

30. T   F   When you enter the room of a client with contact precautions, you should never wear gloves.

MULTIPLE RESPONSE

From the list below, choose all of the correct answers.

31. What are some common signs and symptoms of a systemic infection?
    A. Redness in the area
    B. Swelling of the area
    C. Complaints of pain or tenderness
    D. Low body temperature
    E. Chills
    F. Decreased pulse
    G. Increased respiratory rate
    H. Fatigue and loss of energy
    I. Increased appetite
    J. Discharge from the infected area that may have a foul odour

32. Nancy is a support worker caring for a client in the home. She should wash her hands:
    A. Approximately one half hour before and after giving care
    B. Only when the hands are visibly soiled
    C. After contact with her own or another's blood, body fluids, secretions, or excretions
    D. After touching objects that are contaminated (e.g., soiled linens, garbage bags)
    E. Before and after preparing and handling only foods that must be heated
    F. Before feeding the client
    G. While wearing gloves
    H. After personal body functions (e.g., going to the bathroom, sneezing)

33. What guidelines should be followed when cleaning equipment?
    A. Wear personal protective equipment (PPE) when cleaning items that may be contaminated with blood, body fluids, secretions, or excretions.
    B. Wash the item with soap and bleach.
    C. Scrub the item thoroughly.
    D. Rinse the item in cold water.
    E. Dry the item.

34. Standard Practices are used to prevent the spread of infection from:
    A. Blood
    B. Blood from people who live high-risk lifestyles only
    C. All body fluids, secretions, and excretions (except sweat)
    D. All body fluids, secretions, and excretions (including sweat)
    E. Non-intact skin (skin with open breaks)
    F. Mucous membranes

35. You should allow a client to see your face before you put on personal protective equipment:
    A. Because children may be afraid if they cannot see your face
    B. Because clients with confusion or dementia may be afraid if they cannot see your face
    C. To avoid clients thinking you are there to rob them

36. Aseptic measures the support worker can use in the health care facility to control the transmission of infection include:
    A. Assisting clients with handwashing as necessary
    B. Washing hands properly morning, afternoon, and evening
    C. Cleaning, disinfecting, and sterilizing equipment, as appropriate
    D. Maintaining personal hygiene
    E. Keeping vaccinations up to date

    F. Keeping tables, countertops, wheelchair trays, and other surfaces clean and dry
    G. Washing contaminated areas with tap water
    H. Providing for the client's skin care and oral hygiene, according to the care plan
    I. Covering nose and mouth with a mask when coughing or sneezing
    J. Ensuring clients have their own care equipment, and not sharing items among clients
    K. Taking equipment and supplies from one client's room and using with another client to reduce expenses
    L. Holding equipment and linens close to the body
    M. Covering bedpans and commodes with a lid when transporting
    N. Avoiding sitting on a client's bed
    O. Not using items that have touched the floor for 5 seconds or more
    P. Disinfecting tubs, showers, shower chairs, bedpans, urinals, and commodes after each use

37. When you are assigned to care for a client in isolation, you should tell the nurse if you have:
    A. Tattoos under your uniform
    B. Broken skin on your face, arms, or legs
    C. Fever
    D. Vomiting
    E. Diarrhea
    F. Sore throat
    G. Asthma

38. Types of sharps containers that may be used in home care include:
    A. Containers according to employer policy
    B. Containers that you can easily open to empty
    C. Containers that are puncture-resistant
    D. Containers that are leakproof

39. When you care for a client with an infection, what precautions should be used when handling contaminated laundry?
    A. Sort or rinse linen only in client care area.
    B. Hold soiled linens away from your uniform. Wear gloves.
    C. Remove soiled linens by folding them with the cleanest areas in the centre.
    D. Linen contaminated with blood, body fluids, secretions, or excretions must be placed in a sturdy, leakproof laundry bag labelled with the biohazard symbol.
    E. Bag soiled linen in the room where it was used.

MULTIPLE CHOICE

Circle the correct answer.

40. When your hands are contaminated while working in a health care facility, you should wash them for at least:
    A. 3 to 5 minutes
    B. 2 minutes
    C. 15 to 20 seconds
    D. 1 minute

41. Which of these statements reflects good, aseptic technique?
    A. Take clean, unused equipment from one person's room to another room.
    B. Clean from the dirtiest area to the cleanest area.
    C. Wear protective equipment as needed.
    D. Keep tables and other surfaces clean by wiping them down with the client's facecloth.

42. Here is a list of common aseptic practices that you should use. Which one is the most important to prevent the spread of infection?
    A. Bathing, washing hair, and brushing teeth regularly
    B. Washing cooking utensils with soap and water

C. Covering nose and mouth when coughing or sneezing
    D. Washing hands immediately before and after client care as necessary

43. Transmission-Based Precautions are used:
    A. When caring for all clients
    B. When caring for clients with open wounds
    C. Depending on how the pathogen is spread
    D. Only when caring for clients with a respiratory infection

44. When you are caring for a client who is in isolation, what should you do if you drop clean linens on the floor?
    A. Pick them up and return them to the stack of clean linens.
    B. They are contaminated and should be thrown in the trash.
    C. They are contaminated and should be placed in the dirty linen container.
    D. Use them immediately so they are mixed with clean linens.

45. Paper towels are used in isolation:
    A. To handle contaminated items
    B. Under clean items or objects
    C. To turn faucets on and off
    D. For all of the above

46. Standard Practices should be used:
    A. Only when you think a person has an infection
    B. Only when you are changing soiled linens
    C. Only when you have open skin wounds
    D. When caring for all persons at all times

47. When you are removing gloves after giving care, which part is considered "clean"?
    A. The inside
    B. The outside
    C. Both sides
    D. Neither side

48. When transporting a client who is in isolation, the client should wear a mask:
    A. At all times
    B. Until she reaches the destination
    C. If she is on airborne or droplet precautions
    D. Only while in an elevator

49. Which of the following aseptic measures will control the portal of entry?
    A. Make sure all clients have their own personal care equipment.
    B. Make sure drainage tubes are correctly connected.
    C. Cover your nose and mouth when coughing or sneezing.
    D. Keep drainage containers below drainage sites.

50. If a container is labelled "biohazard," it contains materials that are:
    A. Sterile
    B. Radioactive
    C. Contaminated
    D. Poisonous

51. Which, if any, of these gloves can be reused after cleaning?
    A. Sterile gloves
    B. Disposable gloves
    C. Utility gloves
    D. None of the above

52. Which of the following statements about wearing gloves is correct?
    A. Remove and discard torn or punctured gloves immediately.
    B. Wear the same gloves when giving care to both people in a semi-private room.
    C. Practise hand hygiene while wearing your gloves.
    D. Hand hygiene is not necessary if you wear gloves.

53. When is double-bagging of biohazardous waste necessary?
    A. Any time contaminated items are removed from the client's room
    B. When the client has contact precautions
    C. When materials are contaminated with body fluids
    D. When the outside of the biohazard bag has been contaminated

54. When putting on sterile gloves, which of the following steps is correct?
    A. Lift the second glove by touching only the inside of the glove.
    B. Pick up the second glove by reaching under the cuff with your hand.
    C. Hold the thumb of your first gloved hand away from your second hand as you put on the glove.
    D. Place the glove package below waist height.

55. How can you help to prevent a decrease in self-esteem when a client is in isolation?
    A. Discourage visits by family and friends
    B. Maintain distance between you and the client
    C. Arrange to spend time to visit with the client
    D. Remain in the room only for a short time

FILL IN THE BLANK

Next to each of the following practices, place the letter of the corresponding Transmission-Based Precaution.

A.   *Airborne precaution*
B.   *Droplet precaution*
C.   *Contact precaution*

56. _____   Do not enter the room of a client with measles or chicken pox if you are susceptible to these diseases.

57. _____   Wear a mask when working within 1 m of the client.

58. _____   Wear gloves when entering the room.

59. _____   Keep the door of the room closed.

60. _____   Wear a gown on entering the room if the client is incontinent or has diarrhea.

61. _____   Wear a tuberculosis respirator when entering the room of a client with known or suspected tuberculosis.

62. _____   Wash your hands immediately with an agent specified by the nurse in charge.

CHAPTER 21

Abuse Awareness

TRUE OR FALSE

Circle T for true or F for false.

1. **T   F**   Usually, the time between abusive events gradually shortens.

2. **T   F**   More men than women are abused by spouses.

3. **T   F**   People who are abused often deny the abuse.

4. **T   F**   Slapping a child is not considered abuse.

5. **T   F**   Emotional and physical abuse are the most common types of abuse of older adults.

6. **T   F**   Agism is another cause of abuse.

7. **T   F**   Failing to provide privacy is not a form of abuse.

8. **T   F**   Changes in mental function can cause someone to become sexually abusive.

9. **T   F**   Masturbation may be the result of urinary problems in a confused client.

10. **T   F**   The best way to handle a client who is masturbating in public is to tell the client to stop.

11. **T   F**   You are legally responsible to report child abuse and (in some jurisdictions) abuse within facilities.

12. **T   F**   Sexual harassment is not considered sexual abuse.

13. **T   F**   Abuse is usually triggered by an event related to the victim.

14. **T   F**   People who were abused as children are not likely to abuse their own children because they know what it was like.

15. **T   F**   In most provinces, you do not have to report abuse of older adults to a public authority if it occurs in home care settings.

MULTIPLE RESPONSE

From the list below, choose all of the correct answers.

16. The three phases in the cycle of abuse are:
    A. Tension-building
    B. Trust-building
    C. Abusive
    D. Denial
    E. Bargaining
    F. Honeymoon

17. A person is more likely to be abusive if he or she:
    A. Holds a responsible job
    B. Has problems with alcohol or drugs
    C. Lives alone
    D. Has a mental illness or severe personality flaws
    E. Has been abused as a child
    F. Is going through a period of high stress

18. Certain situations increase the risk of child abuse. They are:
    A. Family crisis
    B. Single-parenting
    C. Isolation
    D. Caring for children with special needs
    E. Extremely high or low intelligence

19. Why do abused older adults choose not to complain about the abuse?
    A. They do not know they are being abused.
    B. They would rather find a lawyer and sue the abuser in court.
    C. They may fear the abuser.
    D. They may not know where or how to get help.
    E. They may fear being forced to move into a facility if the abuser is the primary caregiver.
    F. They may have physical or mental disabilities that prevent them from reporting.

20. Examples of how workers might abuse clients in a facility or home are:
    A. Using restraints inappropriately
    B. Handling the client roughly
    C. Isolating the client
    D. Stealing from the client
    E. Not reviewing the care plan regularly
    F. Not responding to a call for help
    G. Not checking on the client for long periods of time
    H. Leaving the client in soiled linen or clothes

21. What are some examples of abuse that a support worker may encounter from clients?
    A. Swearing, name-calling, and using racial or cultural slurs
    B. Threats
    C. Denial of meal breaks, drinking water, bathroom use, or handwashing facilities
    D. Hitting, pushing, kicking, spitting, biting, pinching, or other physical attacks
    E. Taking too long to eat meals
    F. Inappropriate touching, sexual assault or harassment

22. What can you do when a client is being abusive?
    A. Stay calm, and stand up so as not to be dominated by the client, but stand far enough away so that the person cannot reach you.
    B. Position yourself close to a door, and note the location of call bells, alarms, and other security devices.
    C. Keep your hands free, but do not touch the client.
    D. Listen to the client. Restate what the person says in your own words.
    E. Raise your voice to show your dominance and control over the client.
    F. Tell the client you will get your supervisor to speak to him. If you cannot leave the room, sound the call bell, alarm, or other security device.

G. If you are at a client's home and think you are in danger, leave the house immediately. Go to a safe place, and call your supervisor.

H. If you are at a client's home, do not leave the client alone. Stay and reason with the client.

FILL IN THE BLANK

Next to each example, place the letter that corresponds to the abuse type.

A. *Neglect*
B. *Sexual abuse*
C. *Emotional abuse*
D. *Financial abuse*
E. *Physical abuse*

23. _____ The person has physical injuries (e.g., burns, bumps, cuts, bruises, etc.).

24. _____ The person's behaviour changes when the caregiver (i.e., the potential abuser) leaves or enters the room.

25. _____ Medications are not purchased.

26. _____ The caregiver insists on being present or within hearing distance of all conversations.

27. _____ New injuries appear while older ones are still healing.

28. _____ The person has an intense fear of bathing or perineal care.

29. _____ Personal hygiene is poor (e.g., ingrown nails, untreated sores, matted hair).

30. _____ The person's living conditions are unsafe, unclean, or inadequate.

31. _____ The person has irritation or injury of the thighs, perineum, or breasts.

32. _____ The person has many unpaid bills.

33. _____ The person has signs of poor nutrition and fluid intake (e.g., weight loss, sunken eyes, dry skin).

34. _____ The person may ask for permission to write cheques or spend money.

35. _____ The caregiver often complains about the client.

MULTIPLE CHOICE

Circle the correct answer.

36. If you suspect a client is being abused, you should:
    A. Call the police
    B. Talk to the family
    C. Report it to the nurse
    D. Talk to the client being abused

37. If you are dealing with an agitated or aggressive client, which of these measures would be most helpful?
    A. Talking to the client in a calm manner
    B. Placing your hand on the client's arm to prevent injury
    C. Closing the door so that other people are not upset
    D. Promising the client you will not tell anyone else about her behaviour

38. During the "honeymoon phase" of the cycle of abuse:
    A. The abuser begins to get moodier and stressed
    B. The abuse can escalate easily even if unprovoked
    C. The abuser often blames the victim for the abuse
    D. The abuser is very apologetic for what happened

39. Mrs. Jones is not allowed to go to the bank. Her son insists on handling all of her finances. This is an example of:
    A. Neglect
    B. Physical abuse
    C. Financial abuse
    D. Sexual abuse

40. Mrs. Jones's son insists on changing his mother's incontinence briefs. This might be a sign of:
    A. Neglect
    B. Physical abuse
    C. Financial abuse
    D. Sexual abuse

41. Mrs. Verbrugghe cannot speak English. Her son refuses to translate things for her, especially legal documents, such as the deed to her house. This might be a sign of:
    A. Neglect
    B. Physical abuse
    C. Financial abuse
    D. Sexual abuse

42. You are meeting your client, Mrs. Yil, for the first time in her home. While talking to her, you notice that she is very groggy. What should you do?
    A. Try to wake her up
    B. Notify your supervisor and ask what to do
    C. Look in her cupboards for medication bottles or empty bottles of alcohol
    D. Ask her if you should come back another time when she is more awake

43. You have been supporting Mrs. Yil for several weeks. During that time, you have noticed that Mrs. Yil is very quiet whenever her daughter comes to visit her. You suspect abuse but cannot prove it. What should you do?
    A. Ask Mrs. Yil after her daughter leaves
    B. Ask Mrs. Yil's daughter if she has noticed how quiet her mother is
    C. Telephone the police and make a complaint
    D. Discuss this situation with your supervisor

44. Miss Keys scratches and punches when it is time for her shower. What should you do?
    A. Stay calm and protect yourself
    B. Refuse to bathe Miss Keys
    C. Use silence and ignore her behaviour
    D. Report her behaviour to the nurse in charge

45. When a client is angry and demanding, it is important to:
    A. Ask the nurse to talk to the client
    B. Ignore the client until her behaviour improves
    C. Treat the person with respect and dignity
    D. Tell the client how irritating she is to the staff

46. A term used to describe infants, babies, or children who are below the norms for body weight, growth, or cognitive development is:
    A. Neglected
    B. Failure to thrive
    C. Refusal to grow
    D. Idiopathic weight challenge

MATCHING

Match the correct terms with their definitions.

47. _____ Failure to meet basic needs

48. _____ Misuse of a client's money

49. _____ Force or violence that causes injury

50. _____ Unwanted sexual activity

51. _____ Words or actions that inflict mental harm

A. Sexual abuse

B. Physical abuse

C. Emotional abuse

D. Financial abuse

E. Neglect

Match the different forms of client abuse with the appropriate description.

52. _____ Threatening punishment or deprival of needs

53. _____ Inflicting punishment on the body

54. _____ Kissing, inappropriately touching, or fondling a child

55. _____ Spending a person's money without consent

56. _____ Providing care against a client's wishes

A. Physical

B. Violation of rights

C. Sexual

D. Financial

E. Emotional

CHAPTER 22

Promoting Client Well-Being

TRUE OR FALSE

Circle T for true or F for false.

1. **T   F**   Personal items in a client's space are arranged as the individual prefers.

2. **T   F**   The support worker may throw away any items in the client's space that are in the way.

3. **T   F**   Make sure the client can reach the telephone, television, and light controls.

4. **T   F**   Moving furniture or belongings may be a safety hazard for a client with poor vision.

5. **T   F**   *Distraction* involves creating an image in the mind.

6. **T   F**   Older clients are at greater risk for undetected disease or injury because they have decreased pain sensations.

7. **T   F**   Crying, fussing, and changes in behaviour are normal in infants and young children.

8. **T   F**   Clients aged birth to 1 year and clients 65 years and over will probably need lower room temperatures.

MULTIPLE RESPONSE

From the list below, choose all of the correct answers.

9. Which of the following are factors that affect pain?
   A.   Past experience
   B.   Anxiety
   C.   Nurse pain assessment
   D.   Support from others
   E.   Culture
   F.   Age

10. The nurse needs certain information to assess the client's pain. Which of the following questions could you ask to help gather this information for the nurse?
    A.   Where is the pain?
    B.   How bad is the pain on a scale of 1–30?
    C.   When did the pain start?
    D.   Describe the pain.

11. Which of the following are safety measures used when the client is receiving strong pain medication?
    A. Keep hospital beds in the lowest position.
    B. Provide assistance when client is ambulating.
    C. Keep bed rails up.
    D. Check on the client every 10 to 15 minutes.
    E. Provide a calm, quiet, darkened environment.

12. Which of the following body responses may be signs and symptoms of pain?
    A. Nausea
    B. Increased pulse, respirations, and blood pressure
    C. Dry skin
    D. Sweating
    E. Vomiting

MULTIPLE CHOICE

Circle the correct answer.

13. The call bell should always be positioned:
    A. On the bed rail
    B. Attached to the pillow
    C. Within the client's reach
    D. On the arm of the chair

14. What type of pain is felt suddenly from injury, disease, trauma, or surgery?
    A. Persistent pain
    B. Severe pain
    C. Acute pain
    D. Mild pain

15. How long should you wait to perform procedures after pain medications are given?
    A. 5 minutes
    B. 10 minutes
    C. 30 minutes
    D. 60 minutes

16. What should you do if a client expresses an intention to leave the facility without the doctor's permission?
    A. Try to talk the client out of it
    B. Tell the nurse immediately
    C. Call the doctor to get permission
    D. Let the client leave as it is his choice

17. If you wish to locate an item in a client's closet, you should:
    A. Wait until the client is out of the room to search for it
    B. Tell the client that you must find the item and begin to search
    C. Ask the client for permission to look for the item
    D. Inform the nurse and have her look for the item

18. You are admitting a new client. Which of these situations should be reported to the nurse immediately?
    A. The client complains of pain and appears to be in distress.
    B. The client cries and expresses a desire to go home.
    C. The client has difficulty hearing you.
    D. Both A and B.

19. Mrs. Smith is being admitted to a facility. She wants a family member to stay with her during the admission process. What should you do?
    A. Tell the family member he or she must leave
    B. Tell the nurse
    C. Understand that this is a critical and emotional time for Mrs. Smith and her family and let the family member stay
    D. Address all questions to the family member because he or she can answer more quickly than Mrs. Smith can

20. Which of the following tasks is a support worker's responsibility when discharging a client?
    A. Packing the client's belongings
    B. Teaching the client about a new diet
    C. Making the client an appointment with the doctor
    D. Teaching the client about dressing changes

21. Which of the following statements about pain is NOT true?
    A. Pain is different for each client.
    B. Pain is easy to measure with objective assessments.
    C. Pain means there is damage to body tissue.
    D. You must rely on the client to tell you about the pain.

22. Which of the following statements does NOT describe persistent pain?
    A. Pain lasts longer than 6 months.
    B. Pain is felt at the site and in nearby areas.
    C. Pain may be constant or occur off and on.
    D. Pain remains long after healing occurs.

23. What type of pain occurs when a client has an amputated leg and still feels pain in the missing limb?
    A. Acute
    B. Persistent
    C. Radiating
    D. Phantom

24. If a client is unable to fall asleep, is unable to stay asleep, or awakens easily and cannot fall back to sleep, the client has which of the following conditions?
    A. Sleep deprivation
    B. Insomnia
    C. Sleepwalking
    D. Emotional problems

FILL IN THE BLANK

Indicate whether each of the words below is:

A.   A behaviour that is a sign or symptom of pain

B.   A descriptive word related to pain

25. _____   Aching

26. _____   Throbbing

27. _____   Groaning

28. _____   Restlessness

29. _____   Squeezing

30. _____   Knifelike

31. _____   Dull

32. _____   Irritability

33. _____   Quietness

MATCHING

Match the definition to the term.

34. _____   Absence of mental or physical stress

35. _____   Directing the client's attention away from pain

36. _____   Creating an image in the mind and focusing on it

A.   Guided imagery

B.   Distraction

C.   Relaxation

Match the age group with the correct average amount of sleep required per day.

37. _____ 17-year-old girl   A. 12–14 hours

38. _____ 65-year-old woman   B. 5–7 hours

39. _____ 5-year-old boy   C. 8–9 hours

40. _____ 6-month-old infant   D. 7–8 hours

41. _____ 35-year-old man   E. 11–12 hours

Match the comfort factors with the actions that the support worker can take to control these factors.

42. _____ Adjusting the thermostat in the room   A. Temperature

43. _____ Turning lights down during rest periods   B. Ventilation

44. _____ Emptying bedpans and urinals promptly   C. Noise

45. _____ Opening windows and doors and turning on fans as the client desires   D. Odours

     E. Lighting

46. _____ Talking quietly to staff members

Match the type of pain with the correct description.

47. _____ Pain is felt at the site of tissue damage and in nearby areas.   A. Acute pain

48. _____ Pain is felt suddenly and lasts a short time.   B. Persistent pain

49. _____ Pain is felt in a body part that is no longer there.   C. Radiating pain

50. _____ Pain lasts longer than 6 months.   D. Phantom pain

CHAPTER 23

Body Mechanics: Moving, Positioning, Transferring, and Lifting the Client

TRUE OR FALSE

Circle T for true or F for false.

1. **T F** Log-rolling keeps the spine straight.

2. **T F** When you lift, move, or carry objects, hold them with your arms extended.

3. **T F** When lifting an object from the floor, bend from the waist.

4. **T F** By using two or more people to help a heavy, weak, or very old client move up in bed, you protect only the client from injury.

5. **T F** A turning pad can be an incontinence pad or a folded sheet.

6. **T F** When transferring a client to a chair, choose a chair based primarily on how comfortable the chair will be.

7. **T F** A client lying in bed or sitting in a chair should be repositioned every 3 to 4 hours.

8. **T F** Rubbing of one surface against another is called *friction*.

9. **T F** The way in which body parts are aligned with one another is called *base of support*.

10. **T F** The skin sticking to a surface, causing the muscles to slide in the direction the body is moving, is called *skinning*.

11. **T   F**   Another name for a transfer or safety belt is a *gait belt*.

12. **T   F**   Turning the client as a unit in alignment in one motion is called *body mechanics*.

13. **T   F**   Another name for the back-lying or dorsal recumbent position is the *supine position*.

14. **T   F**   Another name for the side-lying position is the *sideline position*.

15. **T   F**   The semi-sitting position, with the head of the bed elevated 45 to 60 degrees, is called the *Franklin position*.

16. **T   F**   A left-side-lying position in which the upper leg is sharply flexed is called the *Sims' position*.

17. **T   F**   Another word for *posture* is *body mechanics*.

18. **T   F**   A turning sheet or pad is also called a *transfer sheet* or *pad*.

19. **T   F**   Sitting on the edge of the bed is called *edging*.

20. **T   F**   The position in which the client is placed on his abdomen with his head turned to one side is called the *drone position*.

21. **T   F**   A chair used to move clients from one place to another is called a *wheelchair*.

22. **T   F**   You can provide a better base of support for lifting by standing with your legs and feet apart for a wide base of support.

23. **T   F**   Providing a good base of support will help to reduce the risk of injury.

24. **T   F**   When you move a client up in bed, it is important to protect the skin from shaving.

25. **T   F**   You should place the pillow against the headboard when moving a client up in bed to prevent her head from hitting the headboard.

26. **T   F**   The level of the bed should be raised horizontally when the client is being repositioned to reduce the amount of work the support worker has to do.

27. **T   F**   Two staff members work together when raising an older client's head and shoulders to provide more support for clients with fragile bones and joints.

28. **T   F**   A transfer pad is used to keep the bedding neater and to reduce wrinkling.

29. **T   F**   A transfer belt is used on men who have poorly fitting trousers to keep them from falling down.

30. **T   F**   The seat of the wheelchair is padded to promote the client's comfort.

31. **T   F**   Mechanical lifts are used when a client cannot assist with a transfer.

32. **T   F**   The number of staff members needed to transfer a client from the bed to a chair or wheelchair depends on the client's physical abilities and condition.

33. T F The position shown below is called the *Sims' position*.

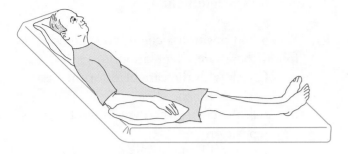

34. T F The position shown below is called the *supine position*.

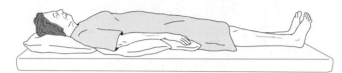

35. T F The position shown below is called the *prone position*.

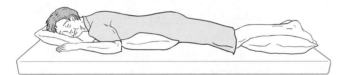

36. T F The position shown below is the *stomach-lying position*.

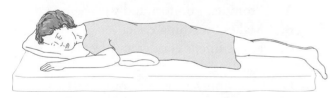

37. T F The position shown below is called the *stroke position*.

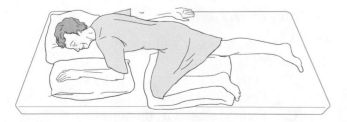

38. T F When lifting correctly, as demonstrated in the figure below, you should use muscles in your shoulders, upper arms, hips, and thighs.

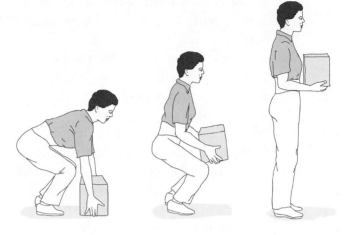

MULTIPLE RESPONSE

From the list below, choose all of the correct answers.

39. When working together, two coworkers can ensure they move the client at the same time by:
    A. One person communicating directions when lifting
    B. Counting to 10
    C. Lifting together

40. It is important for a support worker to follow the guidelines for good body mechanics. They are:
    A. Assess the situation before you begin lifting
    B. Face your work area
    C. Bend your back and squat when lifting
    D. Tighten your stomach muscles and tuck in your pelvis as you lift
    E. Hold objects close to your body when lifting, moving, or carrying them
    F. Avoid unnecessary bending and reaching
    G. Turn your whole body in sections when changing the direction of your movement

41. How can you provide comfort and safety to a client being lifted or moved in bed?
    A. Check with your supervisor and the care plan about limits or restrictions in moving or positioning that client
    B. While you are moving the client, decide how to move the client and how much help you need
    C. Ask for help before starting the move
    D. Communicate directions with your helper by counting 1–2–3, and then moving together
    E. Move the client in one large movement
    F. Cover and screen the client for privacy
    G. Make sure tubes or drainage containers connected to the client are not pulled, tangled, or pinched during the move
    H. Position the client in good alignment after the move
    I. Make sure linens are wrinkle-free after moving the client

42. Log-rolling is used to turn:
    A. Clients with arthritic spines or knees
    B. Clients recovering from hip fractures
    C. Clients with spinal cord injuries
    D. Clients with facial injuries
    E. Clients recovering from spinal cord surgery

43. What observations should you make when the client is dangling the legs?
    A. Pulse and respirations (if instructed to do so)
    B. The length of time the person's legs dangled
    C. Complaints of dizziness, light-headedness, or difficulty breathing
    D. How well the activity was tolerated
    E. The amount of assistance that you wish you had

44. Before using a lift, make sure:
    A. The client has read the lift policy for your agency
    B. You are trained to use the lift
    C. The lift works
    D. The client's weight does not exceed the lift's weight limit

45. When you position a client, you should follow these safety regulations:
    A. Check with the care plan for the best position for the client.
    B. Ask the client when you should reposition her.
    C. Use good body mechanics.
    D. Ask for help before beginning the process.
    E. Explain the procedure to the client after performing the procedure.
    F. Be gentle when moving the client.
    G. Provide for privacy.
    H. Leave the client in good body alignment.
    I. Use pillows as directed in the care plan for comfort and support.
    J. Make sure linens are wrinkle-free by tucking the top sheet under the mattress.
    K. In facilities, place the call bell within the client's reach.

46. What are the benefits of repositioning a client frequently?
    A. Promotes comfort and well-being
    B. Makes breathing easier
    C. Keeps linens cleaner and fresher smelling
    D. Helps prevent many complications (e.g., pressure ulcers and contractures)

MULTIPLE CHOICE

Circle the correct answer.

47. A transfer sheet or pad is used by placing it under the client:
    A. From the head to above the knees
    B. From the shoulders to the hips
    C. From the head to the hips
    D. From the shoulders to the knees

48. Why should shoes with non-skid soles be worn by the client being transferred to a chair or wheelchair?
    A. To provide a good base of support
    B. To make the client more steady on his feet
    C. To prevent the client sliding or slipping on the floor
    D. To provide strength on the client's weak side

49. When transferring a client to a stretcher:
    A. Three or more staff members are needed
    B. A transfer belt is used to lift the client
    C. The head of the stretcher is raised before the transfer
    D. The client is moved by moving the head first

50. *Body alignment* is:
    A. The way the head, trunk, and legs are aligned with each other
    B. The same as *body mechanics*
    C. The base of support
    D. The area on which an object rests

51. The back-lying position is called:
    A. The supine position
    B. Fowler's position
    C. Sims' position
    D. The prone position

52. Miss Polly Walker is lying on her left side. Her upper leg is sharply flexed. This is called:
    A. The supine position
    B. Low Fowler's position
    C. Sims' position
    D. The prone position

53. Miss Polly Walker has the head of her bed elevated 60 degrees. This position is called:
    A. The supine position
    B. High Fowler's position
    C. Sims' position
    D. The prone position

54. Mr. John Dunlop is turned as a unit, with one motion. This is called:
    A. Body mechanics
    B. Log-rolling
    C. Ergonomics
    D. The safety roll

55. Mrs. Renee Nadeau has slid down in bed. Her skin sticks to the bed while her muscles move down. This is called:
    A. Friction
    B. Abrasion
    C. Tension
    D. Shearing

56. When you are giving bedside care, the bed should be:
    A. At its lowest horizontal level
    B. At its highest horizontal level
    C. Level with your waist
    D. In Fowler's position

57. You need to move a client up in bed. To reduce your risk of injury:
    A. Use a transfer sheet
    B. Use a transfer belt
    C. Raise the bed height to waist level
    D. Get assistance from a coworker

58. To prevent falls during transfers, you should ensure that wheelchair or shower chair wheels are:
    A. Fully inflated
    B. Locked and aligned correctly
    C. Removed
    D. Positioned sideways and at right angles to the chair

59. Mrs. Arja Gupta has weakness on her left side. Where should you position the wheelchair?
    A. At the foot of the bed
    B. At the head of the bed
    C. Next to the bed on her left side
    D. Next to the bed on her right side

60. When you have to move, turn, or transfer a client, it is always best to:
    A. Use a transfer belt
    B. Have a coworker help you
    C. Follow the care plan
    D. Use a mechanical lift

61. Before moving, turning, transferring, or lifting a client, you should always:
    A. Explain what you are going to do in a way the client understands
    B. Ask a coworker to help you
    C. Apply a transfer belt
    D. Use a mechanical lift

62. A no-lift policy means:
    A. You should not bend over to pick up something that fell to the floor
    B. Mechanical lifts need to be used for lifting clients
    C. Only the special lift team is allowed to lift clients
    D. Clients are not allowed to be lifted at any time

CHAPTER 24

Exercise and Activity

TRUE OR FALSE

Circle T for true or F for false.

1. **T** **F** Exercise every joint on every client.

2. **T** **F** Support the extremity being exercised.

3. **T** **F** Exercise the joint to the point of pain.

4. **T** **F** The client should wear soft slippers or sandals when using crutches.

5. **T** **F** Loose clothing can hang forward and block the client's view of the feet and crutches.

6. **T** **F** A pouch attached to a walker makes the client more dependent on others.

7. **T** **F** When a client is on bed rest, some ADLs are allowed, such as feeding and oral hygiene.

8. **T** **F** Strict bed rest means everything is done for the client.

9. **T** **F** Bed rest with commode privileges means the client can use the bathroom for elimination needs.

10. **T** **F** Plantar flexion and footdrop can be prevented by using a footboard.

11. **T** **F** A trochanter roll can be used to prevent external rotation of the hips and legs.

12. **T** **F** A hip abduction wedge keeps the hips together.

13. **T** **F** If a client is falling, you should try to stop the fall.

14. **T** **F** When ambulating, the cane is used on the strong side.

15. **T** **F** A walker gives more support than a cane.

MULTIPLE RESPONSE

From the list below, choose all of the correct answers.

16. Which of the following are benefits of bed rest?
    A. Reduces physical activity
    B. Reduces pain
    C. Reduces pressure ulcers
    D. Encourages rest
    E. Promotes healing

17. Which of the following is correct when a client is using a cane?
    A. The cane is used on the weak side.
    B. The client should move the cane forward 15–25 cm at a time.
    C. The client should move the strong leg forward first.

MULTIPLE CHOICE

Circle the correct answer.

18. Which of the following statements correctly describes a type of bed rest?
    A. The client remains in bed but is allowed to perform some activities of daily living (ADLs).
    B. The client can use the bedside commode for elimination needs.
    C. Everything is done for the client; no ADLs are allowed.
    D. All of the above describe bed rest.

19. Which of the following steps would be used to prevent orthostatic hypotension?
    A. Assist the client to lie on the edge of the bed.
    B. Ask the client about weakness, dizziness, or spots before the eyes.
    C. Have the client stand up quickly when getting out of bed.
    D. Measure blood pressure, pulse, and respirations each time the client changes position.

20. Which of the following is a complication of bed rest?
    A. Urinary retention
    B. Diarrhea
    C. Blood clots
    D. Diabetes

21. What is one range-of-motion exercise that a support worker can assist with only if allowed by her agency?
    A. Hip abduction and adduction
    B. Neck exercises
    C. Knee exercises
    D. Shoulder exercises

22. When you move a joint during range-of-motion exercises and the client complains of pain, what should you do?
    A. Ask the nurse to give pain medication before you continue
    B. Do not force the joint to the point of pain
    C. Stop doing any range-of-motion exercises with the client
    D. Push slightly past the point where pain occurs to restore movement

23. When performing range-of-motion exercises, how often should each exercise be repeated?
    A. Once
    B. Twice
    C. Five times or according to the care plan
    D. Until the client complains of being tired

24. Improperly fitted crutches can cause:
    A. Falls
    B. Back pain and nerve damage
    C. Injuries to the underarms and palms
    D. All of the above

MATCHING

Match the following statements with the correct terms related to exercise and activity.

25. _____ Support placed to prevent external rotation of hips and legs

26. _____ Swinging bar on overbed frame that allows the client to move in bed

27. _____ Decrease in size or wasting away of tissue

28. _____ Turning downward

29. _____ Device placed to keep soles of feet flush against it with feet in flexed position

30. _____ Abnormal shortening of a muscle

31. _____ Sections of plywood used to prevent mattress from sagging

32. _____ Footdrop

33. _____ Exercise of all joints of the body

A. Footboard

B. Contracture

C. Atrophy

D. Bed board

E. Plantar flexion

F. Trochanter roll

G. Trapeze

H. Range-of-motion

I. Pronation

Match each movement with the description.

34. _____   Turn head from side to side   A.   Abduction

35. _____   Turn hand so palm is down   B.   Adduction

36. _____   Turn hand toward thumb   C.   Flexion

37. _____   Bend arm so that same-side shoulder is touched   D.   Internal rotation

38. _____   Pull foot forward and push down on heel at same time   E.   Extension

39. _____   Move straight arm away from side of body   F.   Hyperextension

40. _____   Turn foot down or point the toes   G.   Rotation

41. _____   Move head to the right and to the left   H.   Lateral flexion

42. _____   Touch each fingertip to thumb   I.   External rotation

43. _____   Turn hand toward little finger   J.   Pronation

44. _____   Move forearm toward head   K.   Supination

45. _____   Move leg toward the other leg   L.   Opposition

46. _____   Straighten fingers so fingers, hand, and wrist are straight   M.   Plantar flexion

47. _____   Bend the hand back   N.   Dorsiflexion

48. _____   Turn inside of foot up and outside down   O.   Radial flexion

49. _____   Turn leg inward   P.   Ulnar flexion

Match the following types of range-of-motion exercises with the correct definition.

50. _____   Someone moves the client's joints through ROM   A.   Active
               exercises
                                                                      B.   Passive
51. _____   The client does the exercises with the help of another
               person   C.   Active-assisted

52. _____   The client does the exercises by himself

CHAPTER 25

Home Management

TRUE OR FALSE

Circle T for true or F for false.

1. **T**   **F**   Work from dirtiest to cleanest.

2. **T**   **F**   Dust from higher surfaces to lower surfaces.

3. **T**   **F**   Use latex gloves when cleaning.

4. **T**   **F**   It is safe to use any cleaner in the bathroom.

5. **T**   **F**   A client recovering from surgery may need extra cleaning done in the bathroom.

6. **T**   **F**   Baking soda will remove stains.

7. **T**   **F**   Any type of soap can be used in the dishwasher.

8. **T**   **F**   Sort clothing by colours before washing.

9. **T**   **F**   Stained items should be soaked in bleach for 10 minutes before washing.

10. **T**   **F**   It is better to dry clothes in a dryer than to hang them outside.

11. **T**   **F**   It is safe to mix chlorine bleach and ammonia to make a stronger cleaner.

MULTIPLE RESPONSE

From the list below, choose all of the correct answers.

12. To complete home management tasks, you need to use your time wisely. Identify the points below that will help you.
    A. Identify priorities.
    B. Establish a routine.
    C. Use your time well—start with tasks that have a waiting period or run automatically, and then go on to other tasks.
    D. Finish tasks, and put items away.
    E. Set time limits for each task.
    F. If one task takes too long, switch tasks. Watch the clock.
    G. Put the client's needs first.

13. To remove urine stains, you should:
    A. Rinse the stained item in hot water
    B. Soak the item in a solution of 1 L warm water, 2 mL liquid handwashing soap, and 15 mL bleach for 30 minutes
    C. Rinse the item in cool water
    D. Soak the item in a solution of 1 L warm water and 15 mL vinegar for 1 hour
    E. Machine wash the item with chlorine bleach (with permission) and detergent. Dry as usual.

14. Your goal when doing laundry is:
    A. To clean items
    B. Not to damage items
    C. To entertain the client

15. When cleaning kitchens, you should remember the following:
    A. Pour dirty or contaminated liquids down the kitchen sink only.
    B. Use one cloth for counters, another for wiping floors, and another for dishes.
    C. Use dishcloths to dry your hands.
    D. Change cloths daily as needed. Wash in bleach and hot water.
    E. Use paper towels for all tasks when possible.
    F. Clean the microwave inside and out after every use.
    G. Do not put soiled diapers into the kitchen garbage.

16. What can you do to decrease microbes in the bathroom?
    A. Remove and dispose of hair from the sink, tub, or shower.
    B. Flush the toilet with the seat down to prevent splashing.
    C. Rinse the sink after it has been used for washing, shaving, or oral hygiene.
    D. Hang damp towels and bath mats up to dry. Spread them out.
    E. Wash bath mats, the wastebasket, and the laundry hamper every week.
    F. Close shower doors.
    G. Let the bathtub or shower drip dry after use.
    H. Flush dirty or contaminated liquids down the toilet only.

17. Cleaning products can cause harm if not used properly. Remember to:
    A. Read all labels carefully
    B. Never mix cleaning products
    C. Wear latex gloves
    D. Never use products in unlabelled containers
    E. Store products in their original containers
    F. Keep cleaning products away from food
    G. Keep cleaning products out of reach of children and of adults with dementia
    H. Use products only for their intended purpose
    I. Keep aerosol cans away from heat sources
    J. Ask the client before using a strong cleaner on a surface
    K. Rinse away strong, abrasive cleaners immediately after use
    L. Scrub vigorously when cleaning

18. What are some general cleaning guidelines?
    A. Clear away clutter.
    B. Work from lower to higher.
    C. Work from near to far.
    D. Work from dry to wet.
    E. Work from dirtiest to cleanest.
    F. Change cloths and water frequently.
    G. Use a dry cloth for dusting.
    H. Rinse and dry washed surfaces.
    I. Avoid soiling a clean area.

MULTIPLE CHOICE

Circle the correct answer.

19. When should spills and splashes be cleaned up?
    A. After meals
    B. Weekly
    C. Before you leave for the day
    D. Immediately

20. Which statement about laundry care is true?
    A. All clothing should be ironed.
    B. All whites should be washed together.
    C. All whites are washed in hot water.
    D. Care label instructions should be followed.

21. You notice the client's clothing is missing care labels. What should you do?
    A. Ask the client for washing guidance.
    B. Guess how each article should be washed.
    C. Wash everything by hand.
    D. Wash everything in cold water.

22. Why should cleaning products never be mixed together?
    A. Mixing chemicals reduces their cleaning effect.
    B. Cleaners may become toxic if mixed.
    C. Mixed chemicals can stain your hands.
    D. They might make the article dirtier.

23. Which statement on food handling is true?
    A. Always wear gloves while cooking.
    B. Garbage should be disposed of weekly.
    C. Leftover food should be refrigerated immediately.
    D. Season the client's food to your taste.

MATCHING

Match each laundry symbol to its meaning.

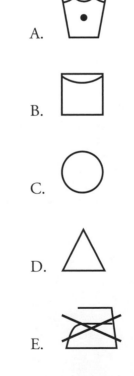

24. _____ Dry clean.   A.

25. _____ Handwash gently in cool water.   B.

26. _____ Machine-wash in hot water.   C.

27. _____ Use chlorine bleach with care.   D.

28. _____ Do not iron or press.   E.

29. _____ Hang to dry after removing excess water.   F.

CHAPTER 26

Beds and Bed Making

TRUE OR FALSE

Circle T for true or F for false.

1. **T** **F** In long-term care, an open bed is made because most clients are out of bed all day.

2. **T** **F** Clients in long-term care facilities may use their own linens.

3. **T** **F** If a client receiving home care refuses to have his linens changed, you should follow the client's wishes.

4. **T** **F** The space between the mattress and crib sides should be no more than 5 cm (2 in.).

5. **T** **F** A surgical bed is made by fanfolding the linens to the side of the bed closest to the door.

6. **T** **F** Shaking bed linens spreads microbes.

7. **T** **F** Making one side of the bed before going to the other saves the support worker time and energy.

MULTIPLE RESPONSE

From the list below, choose all of the correct answers.

8. What are some of the disadvantages of using a plastic drawsheet?
   A. Plastic drawsheets retain heat.
   B. Plastic drawsheets may make the client uncomfortable.
   C. Plastic drawsheets are hard to keep tight and wrinkle-free.
   D. Plastic drawsheets used on the bed may protect the mattress and bottom linens from dampness and soiling.

9. When you are making an occupied bed, which of the following are concerns you should have about the client in the bed?
   A. Make sure the client is in good body alignment.
   B. Know about restrictions or limitations concerning the client's movement or positioning.
   C. Make sure the client is out of the bed.
   D. Make sure that you explain each step of the procedure to the client.

10. What are the five basic bed positions?
    A. Fowler's position
    B. Reverse Fowler's position
    C. Trendelenburg's position
    D. Reverse Trendelenburg's position
    E. Semi-Trendelenburg's position
    F. Semi-Fowler's position
    G. Flat

MULTIPLE CHOICE

Circle the correct answer.

11. When you are changing bed linens, when should you wear gloves?
    A. At all times
    B. When linens are soiled with blood, body fluids, or body secretions or excretions
    C. When you are handling the clean linens
    D. Before the client has had a bath

12. Which statement is true when you are making an occupied bed?
    A. The client gets up and sits in a chair while you make the bed.
    B. You must keep the client in good alignment while making the bed.
    C. The top linens are folded so that a client can be transferred from a stretcher to the bed easily.
    D. The occupied bed is made after a client is discharged from the facility.

13. Why do you raise the level of the bed when you are changing linens?
    A. So that you can use good body mechanics to prevent injury
    B. To prevent injury to the client in bed
    C. To allow space under the bed for cleaning
    D. So that you can keep the client in good body alignment

14. Which bed position is used after a spinal cord injury?
    A. Semi-Fowler's
    B. Flat
    C. Trendelenburg's
    D. Fowler's

15. Which statement is true?
    A. Shake the sheets to get rid of crumbs.
    B. Do not tuck the top sheet under the mattress.
    C. Put dirty linens on the floor.
    D. Hold linens away from your uniform.

MATCHING

Match each term with the correct definition.

16. _____ Closed bed

17. _____ Open bed

18. _____ Occupied bed

A. Top linens are folded for transferring the client to or from a stretcher

B. A bed made with the client in it

C. Top linens are pulled up and the bedspread is pulled neatly over the pillow

You are getting ready to change bed linens. Number the linens you collect in the correct order from 1 to 9.

19. _____ Bedspread

20. _____ Plastic drawsheet

21. _____ Bottom sheet

22. _____ Bath blanket

23. _____ Cotton drawsheet

24. _____ Mattress pad

25. _____ Top sheet

26. _____ Pillowcases

27. _____ Blanket

CHAPTER 27

Nutrition and Fluids

TRUE OR FALSE

Circle T for true or F for false.

1. T   F   The body becomes swollen if too much sugar is retained.

2. T   F   When a healthy client eats more sodium than the body needs, it will be excreted.

3. T   F   A client with diabetes will retain salt in the body.

4. T   F   When a client has diabetes, sugar builds up in the bloodstream.

5. T   F   When a client is placed on a diabetic diet, only three meals each day are allowed.

6. T   F   A client on a clear-liquid diet is allowed water, gelatin, and popsicles.

7. T   F   A client who has constipation may be helped by a high-fibre diet.

8. T   F   Many special diets involve between-meal nourishments such as crackers and milk.

9. T   F   There are four calories in 1 g of carbohydrate.

10. T   F   One gram of fat contains nine calories.

11. T   F   One gram of protein contains five calories.

12. T   F   Chopped foods may be added to an infant's diet at about 5 months of age.

13. T   F   Beef is generally not eaten in India.

14. T   F   Clients who must eat in bed should be positioned in the supine position.

15. T   F   A decrease in saliva may cause difficulty swallowing.

16. T   F   Decreased peristalsis results in slower emptying of the stomach and colon, causing flatulence and constipation.

17. T   F   Cooked fruits and vegetables may be eaten to prevent constipation.

18. T   F   Too much sodium in the diet causes the body to retain more water.

19. T   F   When a client is on a sodium-restricted diet, the only food group without restrictions is fruits and vegetables.

20. T   F   The client with diabetes must eat at regular times to maintain her cholesterol levels.

21. T   F   When a client has dysphagia, the care plan might indicate that he is on a pureed diet.

22. T   F   The daily minimum amount of water required for an adult to survive is 800 mL.

23. T   F   To maintain normal fluid balance, a client needs 2000–2500 mL each day.

24. T   F   An older client should increase calorie intake, as more calories are needed as we age.

25. T   F   An older client should increase fluid intake to aid in digestion, kidney function, chewing, and swallowing.

26. T   F   An older client should increase protein intake for tissue growth and repair.

27. T   F   An older client should decrease soft bulk to prevent constipation.

28. T   F   An older client should decrease intake of fried, fatty foods as these are hard to digest.

MULTIPLE RESPONSE

From the list below, choose all of the correct answers.

29. Which of the following dietary guidelines are recommended for healthy eating?
    A.   Select dietary choices only from one food group.
    B.   Emphasize cereals, breads, other grain products, vegetables, and fruit.
    C.   Choose higher-fat dairy products, leaner meats, and foods prepared with little or no fat.
    D.   Participate in regular physical activity and healthy eating.
    E.   Limit salt, alcohol, and caffeine.

30. In what ways, other than positioning, can you help a client to get ready for meals?
    A.   Assist with elimination and hand hygiene.
    B.   Change clothing and provide clean linens if necessary.
    C.   Be sure dentures, eyeglasses, and hearing aids are in place.
    D.   Decide their menu choices.
    E.   Make the setting attractive.

31. Which of the following actions are important for safety and comfort when feeding a client?
    A.   Provide a relaxed mood.
    B.   Provide time and privacy to pray.
    C.   Use a fork to feed the client.
    D.   Offer larger portions.
    E.   Offer fluids during the meal.
    F.   Engage the client in conversation.
    G.   Stand while you are feeding your client.
    H.   Encourage your client to feed herself.

32. Which of the following are common causes of dehydration?
    A.   Adequate fluid intake
    B.   Vomiting
    C.   Diarrhea
    D.   Bleeding
    E.   Excess sweating
    F.   Decreased urine production

33. Which of the following food groups are included in *Eating Well with Canada's Food Guide*?
    A. Grain products
    B. Vegetables and fruit
    C. Sugar and other sweets
    D. Milk products
    E. Meat and alternatives

MULTIPLE CHOICE

Circle the correct answer.

34. Why are carbohydrates important in the diet?
    A. They supply products for tissue growth and repair.
    B. They provide energy and bulk for bowel elimination.
    C. They provide energy and flavour.
    D. They supply vitamins that are needed daily.

35. What can you give a client who has an order for NPO?
    A. Unlimited fluids
    B. No food or fluids
    C. Small amounts of fluids
    D. Only clear liquids

36. What effect may cultural and religious beliefs have on nutrition?
    A. Certain types of food may be restricted.
    B. Methods of preparation may be part of beliefs.
    C. Certain foods are eaten, and others are avoided.
    D. All of the above may be part of beliefs.

37. Which of these foods would not be included as liquid intake?
    A. Tomato soup
    B. Cream of wheat cereal
    C. Beef vegetable soup
    D. Chocolate pudding

38. Which of the following statements describes assistive dining?
    A. One client is fed by one support worker to reduce stimulation.
    B. Food is placed on platters or dishes, and the clients serve themselves.
    C. Clients are served food at the table as in a restaurant.
    D. Four clients are seated at a horseshoe-shaped table and are fed by one support worker.

Use the following conversion table to answer questions 39 to 46.

1 oz = 30 cc (mL)
1 cup = 240 cc (mL)
1 quart = 1000 cc (mL)
1 cc = 1 mL

39. A 6-oz cup of coffee = how many cc's?
    A. 160 cc
    B. 180 cc
    C. 170 cc
    D. 200 cc

40. 8 oz of milk = how many cc's?
    A. 200 cc
    B. 260 cc
    C. 240 cc
    D. 230 cc

41. 1 quart of water = how many cc's?
    A. 1000 cc
    B. 900 cc
    C. 1020 cc
    D. 1010 cc

42. 2 cups of tea = how many cc's?
    A. 460 cc
    B. 440 cc
    C. 480 cc
    D. 400 cc

43. 4 oz of gelatin = how many cc's?
    A. 100 cc
    B. 120 cc
    C. 130 cc
    D. 140 cc

44. 5 oz of orange juice = how many cc's?
    A. 150 cc
    B. 130 cc
    C. 170 cc
    D. 140 cc

45. 12 oz of broth = how many cc's?
    A. 340 cc
    B. 380 cc
    C. 360 cc
    D. 320 cc

46. A half-cup of sherbet = how many cc's?
    A. 100 cc
    B. 110 cc
    C. 120 cc
    D. 130 cc

MATCHING

Match the nutrient with the reason it is important to good health.

47. _____   Needed for tooth and bone formation

48. _____   Needed for tissue growth and repair

49. _____   Provides energy and adds flavour

50. _____   Provides energy and fibre for elimination

51. _____   Does not provide calories but is needed for certain body functions

A. Protein

B. Carbohydrates

C. Fats

D. Vitamins

E. Minerals

Match the vitamin with its major function.

52. _____   Healthy eyes, healthy skin and mucous membranes, protein and carbohydrate metabolism

53. _____   Formation of substances that hold tissues together

54. _____   Formation of red blood cells, nervous system functioning

55. _____   Blood clotting

56. _____   Normal reproduction

57. _____   Growth, vision, healthy hair and skin

58. _____   Muscle tone, nerve function, digestion

59. _____   Protein, fat, and carbohydrate metabolism

60. _____   Formation of red blood cells, functioning of intestine

61. _____   Absorption and metabolism of calcium and phosphorus, healthy bones

A. Vitamin A

B. Thiamine

C. Riboflavin

D. Niacin

E. Vitamin B_{12}

F. Folic acid

G. Ascorbic acid

H. Vitamin D

I. Vitamin E

J. Vitamin K

Match the mineral with its major function.

62. _____ Formation of bone and teeth; use of protein, fats, and carbohydrates

63. _____ Thyroid gland function, growth, metabolism

64. _____ Fluid balance, nerve function, muscle function

65. _____ Formation of bone and teeth, blood clotting, muscle contraction

66. _____ Enabling red blood cells to carry oxygen

67. _____ Nerve function, muscle contraction, heart function

A. Calcium

B. Phosphorus

C. Iron

D. Iodine

E. Sodium

F. Potassium

Match the appropriate special diet to the following situations.

68. _____ First diet after surgery

69. _____ Constipation and colon disorders

70. _____ Weight gain and certain thyroid imbalances

71. _____ Heart disease, gallbladder disease

72. _____ Burns, high fever, infection

A. High-protein

B. Fat-controlled/low-cholesterol

C. Clear-liquid

D. High-calorie

E. High-fibre

Match the correct food group to the following food items.

73. _____ Crackers

74. _____ Kidney beans

75. _____ Potatoes

76. _____ Ice milk

77. _____ Chocolate bar

A. Vegetables and fruit

B. Grain products

C. Meat and alternatives

D. Milk products

E. Other foods

Match the correct food group to the following food items.

78. _____ Pineapple chunks   A.   Vegetables and fruit

79. _____ Peanut butter   B.   Grain products

80. _____ Oatmeal   C.   Meat and alternatives

81. _____ Butter tart   D.   Milk products

82. _____ Sour cream   E.   Other foods

CHAPTER 28

Enteral Nutrition and Intravenous Therapy

TRUE OR FALSE

Circle T for true or F for false.

1. **T** **F** During a scheduled tube feeding, 400 mL (13.5 fluid oz) is usually given over 20 minutes.

2. **T** **F** Formula for feeding tubes should be heated.

3. **T** **F** The risk of regurgitation is less with nasointestinal tubes.

4. **T** **F** Mouth care is not important when clients are NPO.

5. **T** **F** An intravenous (IV) site on the back of the hand is in a central venous site.

6. **T** **F** Support workers should check the placement of the feeding tube before each feeding.

7. **T** **F** You should clean the client's nose and nostrils around the feeding tube every 4 to 8 hours.

8. **T** **F** Support workers are responsible for maintaining IV therapy.

9. **T** **F** Notify your supervisor immediately if there is any leaking of fluid from the IV site.

10. **T** **F** Clients should be sitting or in the semi-Fowler's position during tube feedings.

11. **T** **F** Scheduled enteral feedings are usually given four times a day.

12. **T** **F** Continuous enteral feedings require an electric feeding pump.

13. **T   F**   When a client is receiving an enteral feeding, he or she is in a supine position for at least 1–2 hours.

14. **T   F**   Frequent oral care can help a client with a feeding tube feel more comfortable.

15. **T   F**   The left-side-lying position should be avoided when a client is receiving enteral nutrition as this position prevents the stomach from emptying.

MULTIPLE RESPONSE

From the list below, choose all of the correct answers.

16. What conditions may require a client to have a feeding tube?
    A.   Cancers of the head, neck, and esophagus
    B.   Coma
    C.   Dysphagia caused by paralysis
    D.   Trauma or surgery to the face, head, mouth, or neck
    E.   Dementia

17. What can cause the feeding tube to move?
    A.   Coughing
    B.   Sneezing
    C.   Vomiting
    D.   Talking
    E.   Suctioning
    F.   Poor positioning

18. When you care for a client with a feeding tube at home, which of the following is the support worker allowed to do?
    A.   Insert feeding tubes.
    B.   Test the position of the tube.
    C.   Give the first dose of a tube feeding.
    D.   Pour formula into a feeding bag.
    E.   Start feed after placement of tube has been verified by the nurse

19. What should be reported to the nurse if the client is receiving a tube feeding?
    A.   Nausea or vomiting
    B.   Discomfort during the tube feeding
    C.   Diarrhea
    D.   Distended abdomen
    E.   Coughing
    F.   Complaints of indigestion or heartburn
    G.   Redness, swelling, drainage, odour, or pain at the ostomy site
    H.   Normal temperature
    I.   Signs and symptoms of respiratory distress
    J.   Complaints of flatulence

20. A client may receive IV therapy to:
    A.   Receive fluids
    B.   Receive minerals and vitamins
    C.   Receive sugar for energy
    D.   Receive blood
    E.   Receive oral medications
    F.   Receive hyperalimentation (a solution highly concentrated with nutrients)

21. What safety measures must be followed when the client has an IV?
    A.   Follow Standard Practices.
    B.   Move the needle or catheter if the IV is not running.
    C.   Follow the safety measures for restraints if the nurse restrains the extremity to prevent the needle or catheter from moving.
    D.   Protect the IV bag, tubing, and needle or catheter when ambulating the client.
    E.   Assist the client with turning and repositioning.
    F.   Move the bag to the side of the bed on which the client is lying, allowing enough slack in the tubing.
    G.   Notify your supervisor immediately if bleeding occurs from the insertion site.
    H.   Notify your supervisor immediately if you notice signs or symptoms of complications.

22. What signs and symptoms indicate that there is a problem with an IV site?
    A. Bleeding
    B. Puffiness or swelling
    C. Pale or reddened skin
    D. Complaints of pain at or above the IV site
    E. Hot or cold skin near the site

23. What signs and symptoms indicate that there is a systemic problem with an IV?
    A. Fever
    B. Itching
    C. Drop in blood pressure
    D. Bradycardia
    E. Regular pulse
    F. Pink skin
    G. Changes in mental function
    H. Loss of consciousness
    I. Difficulty breathing
    J. Increasing urine output
    K. Chest pain
    L. Nausea

MULTIPLE CHOICE

Circle the correct answer.

24. Which of the following describes a gastrostomy tube?
    A. A tube is inserted through a surgical opening into the stomach.
    B. A tube is inserted through the nose and into the stomach.
    C. An opening is made into the middle part of the small intestine.
    D. A tube is inserted through the nose and into the duodenum.

25. What responsibility does the support worker have if a client is being fed through a tube?
    A. Removing the tube after each feeding
    B. Giving clear liquids by mouth
    C. Assisting the nurse in giving feedings
    D. Avoiding giving mouth care

26. Clients who cannot chew or swallow often receive nutrition by:
    A. Enteral nutrition
    B. IV feedings
    C. A liquid diet
    D. A puréed diet

27. Support workers are responsible for:
    A. Inserting feeding tubes
    B. Testing the position of the tube
    C. Giving the first dose of a tube feeding
    D. Providing personal care to the client

28. Physicians order IV therapy to:
    A. Replace minerals and vitamins lost due to illness
    B. Administer medications
    C. Administer blood
    D. All of the above

29. A sign of an IV therapy complication is:
    A. Vomiting
    B. Swelling around the site
    C. Indigestion
    D. Diarrhea

MATCHING

Match the type of feeding tubes with correct gastrointestinal tract route.

30. _____ Gastrostomy tube

31. _____ Percutaneous endoscopic gastrostomy [PEG] tube

32. _____ Jejunostomy tube

33. _____ Nasointestinal tube

34. _____ Nasogastric tube

A. Through the nose into the stomach

B. Through the nose into the small intestine

C. Into the stomach through a surgically created opening

D. Into the intestines through a surgically created opening

E. Into the stomach through a surgically created opening; an endoscope is fed through the mouth and into the stomach

You may care for clients who have IVs in different sites. Match the site where each of these IVs would be inserted.

35. _____ Peripheral

36. _____ Scalp

37. _____ Central venous sites

38. _____ Peripherally inserted central catheter (PICC)

A. In the subclavian vein or the internal jugular vein

B. In the cephalic or basilic veins in the arm

C. On the back of the hand, in the forearm, or in the crease of the elbow

D. On the head

CHAPTER 29

Personal Hygiene

TRUE OR FALSE

Circle T for true or F for false.

1. T   F   Soap dries the skin, especially in older clients.

2. T   F   The support worker decides what skin care products to use when giving a client a bath.

3. T   F   Plain water may be used for the bath when the skin is very dry.

4. T   F   Bath oils and lotions are used to clean the skin.

5. T   F   Adjust the water temperature and pressure before the client gets in the shower.

6. T   F   Illness and disease can cause a bad taste in the mouth.

7. T   F   Some medications and diseases can cause a white coating on the tongue.

8. T   F   Children should learn to brush their teeth at about age 5.

9. T   F   Cold water should not be used to clean or store dentures because it may cause them to warp.

10. T   F   When you are giving mouth care to an unconscious client, it is important to position the client on her back to avoid aspiration.

11. T   F   If an older client with dementia resists your effort to assist with hygiene, you may find ways to work with the client in the care plan.

12. T   F   Older clients with dementia sometimes become agitated and combative during bathing procedures as they do not understand what is happening or why.

13. T   F   The tub or shower should be cleaned before using to prevent the spread of microbes and infection.

14. T   F   The cleanest part of the perineal area is the anal region.

MULTIPLE RESPONSE

From the list below, choose all of the correct answers.

15. When should oral hygiene be performed?
A. Upon awakening
B. After each meal
C. Every other day
D. At bedtime
E. Before meals (if the client wishes)

16. When giving oral care, what observations should you report to the nurse?
A. Dry, cracked, swollen, or blistered lips
B. Redness, swelling, irritation, sores, or white patches in the mouth or on the tongue
C. Bleeding, swelling, or redness of the gums
D. Loose teeth
E. Rough, sharp, or chipped areas on dentures
F. Complaints of pain or discomfort

17. What are reasons for bathing a client?
A. To clean the skin and mucous membranes of the genital and anal areas
B. To remove microbes, dead skin, perspiration, and excess oils
C. To refresh and relax the client
D. To stimulate circulation and exercise body parts

18. How can the support worker help the client with dementia to tolerate a bath?
A. Not rushing the client
B. Using a loud, firm voice
C. Diverting the client's attention
D. Calming the client and trying again later

19. When giving a tub bath or shower, what safety measures will help to prevent falls?
A. Dry the bathroom or shower room floor.
B. Check hand rails, grab bars, hydraulic lifts, and other safety aids to ensure they are in working order.
C. Place a bath mat inside tubs or showers without a non-skid surface.
D. Place needed items out of the client's reach.
E. Place the call bell within the client's reach.
F. Have the client use towel bars when getting in and out of the tub or shower.
G. Do not use bath oils because they make surfaces slippery.
H. Keep bar soap in the dish to prevent the client from slipping on it.
I. Do not leave weak or unsteady clients unattended.
J. Stay within hearing distance if the client can be left alone.

20. What observations should you make and report when you give a client a bath?
A. The colour of the skin, lips, nail beds, and sclera
B. The location and description of rashes
C. Normal skin
D. Bruises or open skin areas
E. Pale or reddened areas, particularly over bony parts
F. Drainage or bleeding from wounds or body openings
G. Swelling of the feet and legs
H. Corns or calluses on the feet
I. Skin temperature
J. Complaints of pain or discomfort

21. What areas are bathed when giving a partial bath?
    A. Face
    B. Hands
    C. Underarms
    D. Feet
    E. Back
    F. Buttocks
    G. Perineal area

22. What are reasons a complete bed bath may be ordered?
    A. The client is conscious.
    B. The client is paralyzed.
    C. The client is in a cast or traction.
    D. The client is weak from illness or surgery.

23. Back massages should not be given to clients with:
    A. Certain heart diseases
    B. Back injuries
    C. Back surgeries
    D. Skin diseases
    E. Some lung disorders

MULTIPLE CHOICE

Circle the correct answer.

24. When giving oral care, why should you wear gloves?
    A. You will have contact with the mucous membranes.
    B. The gums may bleed.
    C. There may be harmful bacteria (pathogens) in the mouth.
    D. All of the above are correct.

25. How often should mouth care be given to an unconscious client?
    A. Once a day
    B. Once each shift
    C. After every meal
    D. Every 2 hours

26. Why should you avoid using bath oils when giving a tub bath or shower?
    A. They make the tub or floor slippery.
    B. They may be irritating to the skin.
    C. They will cause dryness of the skin.
    D. They may collect in skin folds and cause skin breakdown.

27. Before being given a bath, the client should be assisted to the bathroom or offered the commode, bedpan, or urinal because:
    A. This will prevent incontinence during the bath
    B. Bathing stimulates urination
    C. It will prevent skin breakdown during the bath
    D. It will prevent soiling after the bath

28. About how long should a back massage last?
    A. 1 to 2 minutes
    B. 3 to 5 minutes
    C. 6 to 8 minutes
    D. At least 10 minutes

29. What is one reason to provide perineal care at least once a day?
    A. To prevent the growth of microbes that can cause infection
    B. To prevent incontinence
    C. To prevent pain
    D. To provide exercise

30. Which of the following is the correct way to wash the perineal area?
    A. Wash from the anal area toward the urethra.
    B. Wash in a circular motion from the outside to the inside.
    C. Wash from the urethra to the anal area.
    D. Wash back and forth over the entire area several times.

31. When should the bathwater be changed during a complete bed bath?
    A. After washing the chest and abdomen if the water is soapy or cool
    B. Before washing the feet and legs
    C. After giving perineal care
    D. Only if it is soapy or cool

32. Which of these steps is not correct when giving perineal care to a male client?
    A. Retract the foreskin of the uncircumcised male.
    B. Wash the tip of the penis starting at the urethral opening and working outward.
    C. Clean the shaft of the penis with firm, downward strokes.
    D. Leave the foreskin retracted at the end of the procedure.

CHAPTER 30

Grooming and Dressing

TRUE OR FALSE

Circle T for true or F for false.

1. T F How the hair looks has no effect on the client's well-being.

2. T F When brushing hair, start at the scalp and brush to the hair ends.

3. T F If hair is tangled and matted, first start to brush at the scalp and brush to the ends.

4. T F When caring for adolescents, style hair in a manner that pleases the child and parents.

5. T F Older clients need to shampoo more frequently because of decreased oil gland secretion.

6. T F A female client may want you to shave coarse facial hair.

7. T F When you are shaving the face, the client's skin should be loose.

8. T F Fingernails should be trimmed with scissors.

9. T F Brushing and combing are important to prevent tangles in long hair.

10. T F Garbage bags can be used to make a plastic trough to wash the hair of a client in bed at home.

11. T F When you are giving foot care, you should treat corns and blisters.

12. T F Poor circulation to feet and toes can be caused by diabetes or vascular disease.

13. T F Gangrene and amputation are serious complications of foot injuries.

14. T F The best time to clean and trim fingernails is right after they have been soaked or a client has been bathed.

15. T F Shampooing at the sink or on a stretcher is difficult for people with limited range of motion in their legs and hips.

16. T F Standard Practices should always be followed when shaving a client to prevent contact with their blood from a nick or cut.

17. T F An adolescent may need frequent shampooing because oil gland secretion decreases during puberty, resulting in hair that is drier than normal.

18. T F You can soften the skin before shaving by applying a warm towel to the face for a few minutes.

MULTIPLE RESPONSE

From the list below, choose all of the correct answers.

19. What specific measures are needed to comb curly, coarse, or dry hair?
   A. Use a wide-tooth comb.
   B. Wet the hair or use cooking oil to make combing easier.
   C. Begin at the neckline and comb upward, lifting and fluffing hair outward.

20. How can client safety and comfort be achieved with different methods of shampooing?
   A. During a shower or bath, support the back of the client's head with a pillow while shampooing the client's hair.
   B. If the client must lean forward, have him place a folded washcloth over his eyes, and support his forehead with one hand as you shampoo with the other hand.
   C. If the client is in a wheelchair, have her lean back over the sink. Place a folded towel over the sink edge to protect her neck.

D. Make sure the wheelchair is securely locked in place.
E. If the client is on a stretcher, his hair should not be shampooed.
F. If the client is in bed, place a shampoo tray under her head to protect the linens and mattress.

21. If nicks or cuts occur when shaving a client, you should:
   A. Apply direct pressure to the nick or cut
   B. Apply pressure around the nick or cut but never apply pressure directly to the cut itself
   C. Report the nick or cut to your supervisor at once

22. Observations that should be reported to the nurse during foot care include:
   A. Soft, pink, intact skin
   B. Very dry skin
   C. Foot odours
   D. Cracks or breaks in the skin, especially between the toes
   E. Ingrown nails
   F. Loose nails
   G. Reddened, irritated, or calloused areas on the feet, heels, or ankles
   H. No drainage or bleeding
   I. Change in colour or texture of nails, especially black, thick, or brittle nails
   J. Corns, bunions, or blisters

23. When the client requests a shampoo, you should:
   A. Shampoo the client's hair while she is in bed to avoid tiring her out
   B. Follow the client's care plan
   C. Explain that shampooing is not your job
   D. Wear gloves if the client has scalp lesions or head lice

MULTIPLE CHOICE

Circle the correct answer.

24. Microbes (or bacteria) can be found on dirty:
    A. Shoes
    B. Socks
    C. Feet
    D. All of the above

25. A client has long hair. Which procedure cannot be done?
    A. Daily brushing and combing
    B. Shampooing
    C. Cutting the hair to remove tangles and matting
    D. Braiding or styling

26. A female client in a long-term care facility has her hair done weekly at the beauty shop. During her shower, you should:
    A. Wash her hair as usual
    B. Protect her hair with a shower cap
    C. Be careful not to get water on her hair
    D. Wrap a towel around her head to protect her hair

27. Which of these should you wear when you are shaving a client?
    A. Gown
    B. Gloves
    C. Mask
    D. Gown, gloves, and mask

28. Which of these statements is correct about dressing or undressing a client?
    A. Remove clothing from the affected side first.
    B. Put clothing on the affected side first.
    C. Put clothing on the unaffected side first.
    D. Remove clothing from the side farthest away from you first.

29. Which of these steps is correct when you change a gown of a client receiving intravenous (IV) therapy?
    A. Remove the gown from the arm with the IV first.
    B. Gather up the sleeve of the arm with the IV and slide it over the IV site and tubing.
    C. Turn off the IV and disconnect it temporarily while changing the gown.
    D. Put the gown on the arm without the IV first.

MATCHING

Match the words related to personal care with the descriptions below.

30. _____ Excessive body hair

31. _____ Infestation with lice in the pubic area

32. _____ Hair loss

33. _____ An infestation with lice

34. _____ You may groom hair in this manner with the person's permission

35. _____ Excessive amounts of dry, white flakes from the scalp

36. _____ Parasites that can live on different parts of the body

37. _____ You must never do this to matted or tangled hair

38. _____ Infestation of the scalp with lice

39. _____ Infestation of the body with lice

A. Cutting

B. Pediculosis pubis

C. Hirsutism

D. Pediculosis capitis

E. Dandruff

F. Pediculosis

G. Alopecia

H. Pediculosis corporis

I. Lice

J. Braiding

Number the following steps for undressing a client from 1 to 6 to identify the order in which they should be done.

40. _____ Remove pullover garments from the unaffected side, then from the affected side.

41. _____ Remove garments that open in the front from the unaffected side, then from the affected side.

42. _____ Cover the client with a blanket or sheet.

43. _____ Undo buttons, zippers, or ties on garments that open in the front.

44. _____ Remove pants or slacks.

45. _____ Remove garments that open in the back from the unaffected side, then from the affected side.

CHAPTER 31

Urinary Elimination

TRUE OR FALSE

Circle T for true or F for false.

1. **T** **F** When assisting with normal elimination, you should practise surgical asepsis and Standard Practices.

2. **T** **F** Normal elimination is easier if a man can stand or a woman can sit or squat.

3. **T** **F** If a client has osteoporosis, painful joints from arthritis, or a hip replacement, a regular bedpan will be the most comfortable.

4. **T** **F** Incontinence is a common reason for seeking long-term care for a family member.

5. **T** **F** When collecting a specimen, you should use a sterile container.

6. **T** **F** A specimen container must be labelled with the client's initials, room and bed number (if in a facility), date, and time.

7. **T** **F** When you collect a urine specimen, you should tell the client not to have a bowel movement or place toilet tissue in the container.

8. **T** **F** The specimen container and requisition slip are taken to the laboratory in a plastic cup.

9. **T** **F** An adult normally produces 2500 mL of urine every day.

10. **T** **F** A urinal has a hooked handle so it can be passed easily to the client.

11. **T** **F** When you leave a client alone to void, you should place the call bell and toilet tissue within reach.

12. **T** **F** After a client has voided, you should provide perineal care as needed and have the client wash his or her hands.

13. **T** **F** You wear gloves when emptying a bedpan or urinal to avoid contact with urine or stool.

14. **T** **F** If a urinary drainage bag is lower than the bladder, urine can flow back into the client's bladder and an infection can develop.

15. **T** **F** Adhesive tape should never be used to secure a condom catheter because this type of tape does not stretch, and its lack of elasticity might cause blood flow to the penis to be restricted.

16. **T** **F** When securing a condom catheter in place, tape should be applied in a vertical manner on the client's penis.

17. **T** **F** The goal of bladder training is voluntary control of urination.

18. **T** **F** When collecting a midstream urine specimen, you pass the specimen container into the urine stream (or flow) at any point during urination.

19. **T** **F** To prevent the growth of micro-organisms, place a 24-hour urine specimen on ice or in a refrigerator.

20. **T** **F** Urine is strained to see if it contains crystals.

MULTIPLE RESPONSE

From the list below, choose all of the correct answers.

21. Who may use a fracture (bed)pan?
    A. Clients in casts
    B. Clients who do not like to walk to the toilet
    C. Clients with casts on their ankles
    D. Clients with limited back motion
    E. Clients with fragile bones or painful joints
    F. Clients who have recently fractured a hip

22. If a client is embarrassed about voiding with others close by, what can be done to mask the sounds?
    A. Run some water in a nearby tap
    B. Move the client to another floor or ward
    C. Flush the toilet
    D. Play music nearby

23. How can you promote relaxation and not rush the client who is voiding?
    A. Have the client practise meditation while voiding
    B. Talk to the client to provide some diversion
    C. Offer the person something to read
    D. Allow the person enough time to void

24. What measures can you take to help clients with urinary incontinence?
    A. Answer all calls for assistance promptly
    B. Encourage urination at scheduled intervals
    C. Follow the client's bladder training program
    D. Encourage the client to wear clothing with zippers and laces
    E. Encourage the client to do pelvic muscle exercises, as directed by the care plan
    F. Decrease fluid intake before bedtime
    G. Provide good skin care once a day
    H. Provide dry garments and linens
    I. Observe for signs of skin breakdown.
    J. Use incontinence products as directed by the care plan.

25. Urinary tract infections can sometimes be prevented by:
    A. Providing adequate food for the client to eat
    B. Encouraging the client to add bath oil to the tub bath
    C. Instructing the client to wear cotton undergarments
    D. Providing perineal care as needed

26. What disorders and other conditions may cause urinary incontinence?
    A. Urinary tract infections
    B. Menopause
    C. Nervous system disorders
    D. Bladder cancer
    E. Diabetes
    F. Hearing loss

27. Causes for urinary incontinence include:
    A. A weakened pelvic floor
    B. An enlarged prostate
    C. Some medications
    D. Immobility
    E. The use of restraints
    F. Unanswered calls for help
    G. Confusion
    H. Certain surgeries

28. What complications can occur when a client has incontinence?
    A. Skin irritation
    B. Confusion
    C. Skin breakdown
    D. Infection

MULTIPLE CHOICE

Circle the correct answer.

29. Why is voiding in a bedside commode easier than voiding in a bedpan?
    A. It allows for a more normal position for elimination.
    B. It provides more privacy.
    C. It is more comfortable.
    D. It allows the bladder to empty completely.

30. Which of the following correctly describes catheter care?
    A. Wash the perineal area and avoid touching the catheter.
    B. Clean the meatus and the catheter with an alcohol swab.
    C. Clean the catheter from the meatus and down the catheter about 10 cm (4 in.) with soap and water.
    D. Clean the catheter with soap and water, starting about 10 cm (4 in.) below the meatus and washing toward the perineal area.

31. When applying a condom catheter, you should use:
    A. Sterile technique
    B. Standard Practices
    C. Contact precautions
    D. Droplet precautions

32. When a client is having a 24-hour urine specimen collected, what should you do with the first voiding?
    A. Discard it.
    B. Send it to the laboratory.
    C. Place it in the large container used for saving the urine.
    D. Test it for sugar and ketones.

33. Which of these actions would not be helpful in getting a client to void?
    A. Pulling the curtains and closing doors while the client is urinating
    B. Standing next to the bed and talking quietly to the client who is urinating
    C. Running water in the sink while the client is sitting on the toilet
    D. Standing outside the curtain or bathroom door while the client is urinating

34. When emptying a urinary drainage bag, you maintain medical asepsis by:
    A. Using sterile gloves
    B. Placing the measuring container on a paper towel
    C. Placing the measuring container on the overbed table and stooping to read it accurately
    D. Doing all of the above

35. When straining urine, what should you do if you see particles in the strainer?
    A. Place the strainer in the container and send it to the laboratory
    B. Show it to the nurse and then discard it
    C. Send the urine and strainer to the laboratory
    D. Keep the strainer in the client's room until the doctor arrives

36. When using a reagent strip to test urine, the support worker should:
    A. Send the specimen and reagent strip to the laboratory
    B. Ask the nurse to read the strip
    C. Follow the manufacturer's instructions on the container
    D. Teach the client to read the strips

MATCHING

Match each group of words with the effect that it has on urine.

37. _____ Coffee, tea, alcohol

38. _____ Diet high in salt

39. _____ Beets, blackberries

40. _____ Carrots, sweet potatoes

41. _____ Asparagus

A. Cause bright yellow urine

B. Causes a change in urine odour

C. Increase urine production

D. Cause red-coloured urine

E. Decreases urine production

Match each word with its meaning.

42. Painful or difficult urination

43. Blood in the urine

44. Production of abnormally large amounts of urine

45. Scant amount of urine (less than 500 mL in 24 hours)

46. Frequent urination at night

47. An artificial opening between the ureter and the abdomen

A. Polyuria

B. Ureterostomy

C. Oliguria

D. Dysuria

E. Hematuria

F. Nocturia

CHAPTER 32

Bowel Elimination

TRUE OR FALSE

Circle T for true or F for false.

1. **T**   **F**   Feces move through the intestine by a process called *defecation*.

2. **T**   **F**   Constipation is a condition in which bowel movements are less frequent than usual.

3. **T**   **F**   Liquid feces seeping from the anus is not a sign of fecal impaction.

4. **T**   **F**   Fewer than 10 wet diapers per day from an infant may indicate dehydration.

5. **T**   **F**   Enemas can be dangerous.

6. **T**   **F**   A support worker is allowed to insert rectal tubes to relieve flatulence.

7. **T**   **F**   A stoma is painful when touched.

8. **T**   **F**   A client with an ostomy pouch can wear normal clothes.

9. **T**   **F**   When internal bleeding is suspected, feces are checked for blood.

10. **T**   **F**   A commercial enema stimulates and distends the rectum.

11. **T**   **F**   Feces become hard and dry when fluid intake is poor.

12. **T**   **F**   The support worker may help to prevent fecal incontinence by promptly responding to all requests for help using the bathroom, bedpan, or commode.

13. **T**   **F**   One of two goals of bowel training is to develop a regular pattern of elimination, thus preventing fecal impaction, constipation, and fecal incontinence.

14. **T**   **F**   When you are helping a client with bowel training, the client is usually encouraged to use the toilet, commode, or bedpan before a meal.

15. **T**   **F**   A suppository is used to stimulate defecation when bowel training is being done.

16. **T**   **F**   Giving an enema is a delegated task.

17. **T   F**   Commercial enemas stimulate and distend the rectum.

18. **T   F**   Only a saline enema may be given to children.

19. **T   F**   The purpose of an ostomy pouch is to collect feces and flatus.

20. **T   F**   An ostomy bag is changed every day and whenever it leaks.

21. **T   F**   An ostomy pouch can be removed and changed when peristalsis is less active. The best time is usually after breakfast.

22. **T   F**   Feces from an ileostomy is especially irritating to the skin because the small intestine contains digestive juices that are very irritating.

23. **T   F**   Occult blood is bright red blood that can be observed in the stool.

MULTIPLE RESPONSE

From the list below, choose all of the correct answers.

24. What should you observe and report when a client has a bowel movement?
    A. Abnormalities in colour
    B. Abnormalities in amount
    C. Abnormalities in consistency
    D. Abnormalities in odour
    E. Abnormalities in shape
    F. Abnormalities in size
    G. Abnormalities in frequency
    H. Complaints of pain

25. What are some signs of fecal impaction?
    A. Abdominal discomfort and swelling
    B. Cramping
    C. A feeling of fullness or pain in the rectum
    D. Nausea or vomiting
    E. Fever
    F. Increased need or decreased ability to urinate
    G. Liquid feces seeping from the anus
    H. Regular bowel movements

26. What are common causes of constipation?
    A. A high-fibre diet
    B. Ignoring the urge to defecate
    C. Decreased fluid intake
    D. Activity
    E. Medications
    F. Aging
    G. Certain diseases

27. Which of the following comfort and safety measures can the support worker use when assisting a client with fecal elimination?
    A. Assist the client to the toilet or commode, or provide the bedpan, as soon as requested.
    B. Provide for privacy (ask visitors to leave the room, close doors, pull privacy curtains, and close window curtains, blinds, or shades).
    C. Make sure the bedpan is cold.
    D. Position the client in a side-lying position.
    E. Allow enough time for defecation. Do not rush the client.
    F. Place the call bell and toilet tissue within reach.
    G. Leave the room if the client is weak or unsteady.
    H. Provide oral care.
    I. Dispose of stool promptly.
    J. Assist the client with hand hygiene after elimination.

28. What symptoms may occur if flatulence is not relieved?
    A. Abdominal cramping or pain
    B. Shortness of breath
    C. Decreased level of consciousness
    D. Swollen abdomen, or "bloating"

29. Which of the following are reasons that enemas are given?
    A. To remove feces
    B. To relieve constipation or fecal impaction
    C. To encourage weight loss
    D. To clean the bowel of feces before certain surgeries or X-ray procedures
    E. To relieve flatulence and intestinal distension

30. How can odour associated with an ostomy pouch be prevented?
    A. By providing good hygiene
    B. By emptying the pouch when it is leaking
    C. By encouraging the client to avoid gas-forming foods
    D. By putting deodorants into the pouch, according to the care plan

MULTIPLE CHOICE

Circle the correct answer.

31. Which of the following will not assist fecal elimination?
    A. Drinking a hot beverage
    B. Using a bedside commode in a semiprivate room
    C. Taking a walk
    D. Reading a book or newspaper

32. Which of these foods would be most likely to stimulate fecal elimination?
    A. Pudding and gelatin
    B. Whole-grain cereals and fruit
    C. Meat and fish
    D. Pretzels and potato chips

33. Mr. Lane, 85, usually has a bowel movement after breakfast. About 45 minutes after having a bowel movement, he wants to go to the bathroom again. The most likely reason for this is:
    A. Older adults lose control over defecation.
    B. Complete emptying of the rectum does not always occur with older adults.
    C. He may have a tumour or other disorder.
    D. He is concerned about becoming constipated.

34. Which of these may kill normal flora in the intestine?
    A. Antibiotics
    B. Laxatives
    C. Pain medications
    D. Enemas

35. What instruction will the nurse likely give if a client has diarrhea?
    A. Withhold all fluids.
    B. Give the client plenty to drink.
    C. Encourage the client to eat as little as possible.
    D. Give the client foods with plenty of fibre.

36. What would an effective nursing action to relieve flatulence?
    A. Giving an enema
    B. Making sure the diet is high in vegetables
    C. Having the client lie flat in bed
    D. Ambulating the client or placing the client in the side-lying position

37. When the nurse inserts a suppository to stimulate defecation, how soon would you expect results?
    A. In about 30 minutes
    B. Immediately
    C. In 2 to 3 hours
    D. In the morning

38. How much solution is usually given to an adult as a cleansing enema?
    A. 500 to 1000 mL (17 to 34 fluid oz)
    B. 400 mL (13.5 fluid oz)
    C. 120 mL (4 fluid oz)
    D. 250 mL (8.5 fluid oz)

39. Which position is best when giving an enema?
    A. Sims' position
    B. Right position
    C. Semi-Fowler's position
    D. Prone position

40. When giving an enema, what should you do if the client complains of abdominal cramping?
    A. Insert the tube 2 cm (0.78 in.) more
    B. Clamp the tubing until the cramping stops
    C. Discontinue the enema and report the cramping to the nurse
    D. Withdraw the tube about 2 cm (0.78 in.)

41. What is the purpose of a rectal tube?
    A. Relief of constipation
    B. Treatment of fecal impaction
    C. Prevention of diarrhea
    D. Relief of flatulence and distension

42. What is the consistency of the stool if a colostomy is near the end of the large intestine?
    A. Liquid
    B. Soft
    C. Formed
    D. Hard and dry

43. Which of these methods would help to prevent skin breakdown around the stoma?
    A. Clean with alcohol wipes.
    B. Use an antiseptic lotion or petroleum jelly on the skin.
    C. Clean the area with water and mild soap as directed by the nurse.
    D. Wipe with tissues until clean.

44. You should wear gloves when testing a stool for occult blood to:
    A. Prevent contact with body fluids and substances
    B. Prevent contaminating the specimen
    C. Maintain a sterile specimen
    D. Prevent contact with chemicals used in the test

MATCHING

Match the colour of stool to corresponding factors that can cause the stool to change colours.

45. Bleeding in the stomach

46. Bleeding in the lower colon or rectum; also, beets

47. A diet high in green vegetables

A. Green

B. Black

C. Red

Match the correct word to each definition.

48. _____ Semi-solid mass of waste products in the colon

49. _____ Introduction of fluid into the rectum and lower colon

50. _____ Artificial opening between the ileum and abdomen

51. _____ Bowel movement

52. _____ Alternating contraction and relaxation of intestinal muscles

53. _____ Surgical creation of an artificial opening

54. _____ Cone-shaped medication that is inserted into a body opening

55. _____ Gas or air in the stomach or intestines

56. _____ Feces that have been excreted

57. _____ Frequent passage of liquid stools

58. _____ Partially digested food and fluids that pass from the stomach to the small intestine

59. _____ The opening of a colostomy or ileostomy

A.   Defecation
B.   Suppository
C.   Diarrhea
D.   Peristalsis
E.   Feces
F.   Ostomy
G.   Enema
H.   Chyme
I.   Flatus
J.   Stoma
K.   Stool
L.   Ileostomy

CHAPTER 33

Rehabilitation Care

TRUE OR FALSE

Circle T for true or F for false.

1. **T**   **F**   A disability does not affect the client's psychological well-being. It is only a physical problem.

2. **T**   **F**   Rehabilitation begins by preventing complications.

3. **T**   **F**   Rehabilitation often takes less time for older clients than for clients in other age groups.

4. **T**   **F**   Health care workers as well as the client and family members are part of the rehabilitation team.

5. **T**   **F**   Once the health care team sets goals for the client, they can never be changed.

6. **T**   **F**   The goal of using a prosthesis is that it should be like the missing body part in function, appearance, or both.

7. **T**   **F**   Rehabilitation can occur in the community as well as in long-term care settings.

8. **T**   **F**   Good skin care is important in rehabilitation as it can prevent further disability and illness.

9. **T**   **F**   An electric toothbrush may make brushing the teeth more difficult for a client who has limited arm movement.

10. **T**   **F**   The home is assessed by the rehabilitation team after a client goes home.

MULTIPLE RESPONSE

From the list below, choose all of the correct answers.

11. Which of the following are goals of rehabilitation?
    A. To restore function as much as possible for each client
    B. To improve a client's functional abilities
    C. To cure diseases
    D. To teach clients new skills
    E. To prevent further disability and illness

12. Examples of orthoses include which of the following?
    A. Splints
    B. Foot support
    C. Transfer belt
    D. Knee and back braces

13. Common health problems requiring rehabilitation include which of the following?
    A. Acquired brain injury
    B. Alcoholism
    C. Amputation
    D. Brain tumour
    E. Poor nutrition
    F. Cerebral palsy
    G. Chronic obstructive pulmonary disease

14. How can you improve the quality of life for a client with a disability?
    A. Allow the client to practise skills in private.
    B. Share information about a client's progress with other clients.
    C. Allow for personal choice whenever possible.
    D. Focus on the positive.
    E. Only offer praise when goals are met.
    F. Never force clients to do more than they are able.
    G. Perform activities of daily living for the client as much as possible.

MULTIPLE CHOICE

Circle the correct answer.

15. An orthotic is:
    A. An artificial replacement for missing body parts
    B. The process of correcting a deformity
    C. An apparatus worn for support
    D. The process of restoring a client to the highest level of functioning possible

16. Rehabilitation:
    A. Is often slow and frustrating
    B. Occurs quickly
    C. Is carried out only in a hospital
    D. Does not involve the family

17. Occupational therapists on the rehabilitation team:
    A. Lead and coordinate rehabilitation
    B. Assess the performance of activities of daily living
    C. Test speech
    D. Coordinate home care

18. Social workers on the rehabilitation team:
    A. Provide counselling
    B. Help with physiotherapy
    C. Coordinate and provide care at every stage
    D. Evaluate strength

19. Which member of the rehabilitation team assesses the client's performance of activities of daily living?
    A. The physiotherapist
    B. The occupational therapist
    C. The case manager
    D. The speech-language pathologist

MATCHING

Match the following words with the correct definitions.

20. _____ Process of restoring a person to the highest possible level of function

21. _____ Self-care activities performed to remain independent

22. _____ Helps a person regain health and strength

A. Activities of daily living

B. Independence

C. Rehabilitation

CHAPTER 34

Mental Health Disorders

TRUE OR FALSE

Circle T for true or F for false.

1. **T F** Aggression follows a progressive cycle even though it seems to happen suddenly.

2. **T F** *Depression* is a type of dementia that is rarely cured.

3. **T F** Aggressive clients should be restrained.

4. **T F** Anxiety is a factor of all mental health disorders.

5. **T F** Only illegal drugs are abused.

6. **T F** Communication is important when caring for persons with mental health disorders.

7. **T F** *Panic* is the highest level of anxiety.

8. **T F** A panic attack occurs suddenly with no obvious reason.

9. **T F** When a panic attack occurs, the client may experience chest pain.

10. **T F** A *phobia* involves intense fear of an object or situation.

11. **T F** Depression is at one extreme of bipolar affective disorder.

12. **T F** In the manic phase of bipolar disorder, the person feels worthless.

13. **T F** Depression in the older adult is rarely overlooked.

14. **T F** Major depression can occur at any age.

15. **T F** *Psychosis* is a mental disorder in which the perception of reality is impaired.

16. **T F** *Delusion* is a form of hallucination.

17. **T   F**   The term *hallucinations* refers to strange beliefs.

18. **T   F**   Schizophrenia affects one's ability to function in all aspects of life.

19. **T   F**   Someone who has schizophrenia has a split personality.

20. **T   F**   The person who has schizophrenia has problems knowing what is real and what is not.

21. **T   F**   Paranoid clients may have a great many religious delusions.

22. **T   F**   A *compulsion* is a persistent thought or desire.

23. **T   F**   An *obsession* is the persistent (or constant) urge to perform an act.

24. **T   F**   People obsessed with the idea that germs are on their hands will often wash their hands repeatedly.

25. **T   F**   If a person believes he or she is the prime minister of Canada, that person is having a delusion of grandeur.

26. **T   F**   The two most common extremes of bipolar affective disorder are anger and mania.

27. **T   F**   An older client has the following symptoms: fatigue, slow or unreliable memory, agitation, and thoughts of death. It may be that the person is suffering from depression.

28. **T   F**   A client with anorexia nervosa craves food. After eating, the person induces vomiting.

29. **T   F**   A person with bulimia takes diuretics to lose weight.

30. **T   F**   A client with schizophrenia may experience delusions and hallucinations.

31. **T   F**   A person with anxiety experiences vague, uneasy feelings and feels a sense of danger or harm.

32. **T   F**   Antisocial personality disorder tends to run in families. A person with this disorder commonly has extreme mood swings and at times feels very sad, lonely, and worthless.

33. **T   F**   Some words commonly used to describe a person with a bipolar affective disorder include *abusive*, *paranoid*, and *irresponsible*.

MULTIPLE RESPONSE

From the list below, choose all of the correct answers.

34. What are some of the causes of mental health disorders?
    A. Biological factors
    B. Extreme intelligence
    C. Childhood trauma or conflict
    D. Social and cultural factors (e.g., poverty, discrimination, social isolation)
    E. Stressful life events (e.g., death of a loved one, divorce)
    F. Poor physical health or disability

35. The various forms of psychotherapy include:
    A. Psychoanalysis
    B. Behaviour therapy
    C. Group therapy
    D. Diet therapy
    E. Family therapy

36. A person suffering from schizophrenia may exhibit the following behaviours:
    A. Psychosis
    B. Delusions
    C. Increased need for sleeping
    D. Hallucinations
    E. Paranoia

37. Signs and symptoms of depression include:
    A. Bloating and flatulence
    B. Feeling sad, "blue," or hopeless
    C. Itchy skin and hives
    D. Irritability
    E. Reduced interest in almost all activities
    F. Significant weight gain or loss, without dieting
    G. Insomnia or too much sleep
    H. Too much or too little motor activity
    I. Fatigue or loss of energy
    J. Feelings of worthlessness or guilt
    K. Strong desire to eat a nonfood substance
    L. Increased ability to concentrate or think
    M. Difficulties making decisions
    N. Recurrent thoughts of death

MULTIPLE CHOICE

Circle the correct answer.

38. Which of these may cause mental health disorders?
    A. Inability to cope with stress
    B. Chemical imbalances in the body
    C. Characteristics inherited from parents
    D. All of the above

39. Which of the following is an example of an unhealthy coping mechanism?
    A. Going for a walk
    B. Exercising
    C. Chain smoking
    D. Having a piece of cake with a meal

40. An older adult may not be diagnosed with depression because:
    A. It rarely occurs in an older adult.
    B. Treatment of physical problems is more important in the older adult.
    C. The older person may be thought to have dementia.
    D. Depression in older adults is usually mild and does not require treatment.

41. Which of these would be present if a person has delusions of persecution?
    A. Seeing, hearing, or feeling something that is not there
    B. Not sleeping or taking time to tend to self-care needs
    C. Believing that one is mistreated, abused, or harassed
    D. Having poor judgement and morals and lacking ethics

42. When a girl has anorexia nervosa, which of these behaviours is she likely to display?
    A. Dieting even though she becomes emaciated
    B. Withdrawing from the world and showing no interest in others
    C. Regressing to the behaviour of a younger child
    D. Having delusions or hallucinations

43. Which of these substances can be abused?
    A. Legal drugs
    B. Illegal drugs
    C. Alcohol
    D. All of the above

44. Which of the following statements about mental health disorders is true?
    A. Defence mechanisms are a symptom of mental illness.
    B. Persons with paranoid personality disorders trust others.
    C. Depression disorders are common in adults only.
    D. Bipolar affective disorder is characterized by extreme mood swings.

45. What is the best response to use when caring for a depressed client?
    A. "Let me tell you a funny story."
    B. "Would you like to talk about it?"
    C. "Cheer up and don't look so sad."
    D. "Don't worry. Everything will be all right."

46. Your client Mr. Wong has extreme suspiciousness of others and experiences hallucinations. Which approach by the staff would be the most threatening to Mr. Wong?
    A. Forthright and honest
    B. Friendly and emotionally detached
    C. Warm and nurturing
    D. Tolerant and reserved

47. Mr. Wong becomes very angry and states that someone has been in his room and has taken his razor. He is swearing and yelling at the staff. Your best response is:
    A. "I don't blame you for being angry."
    B. "That doesn't make any sense. I don't know who would want your razor."
    C. "This happens all the time" and begin to look in his bedside unit.
    D. "This is very upsetting. Can you show me where you usually keep your razor?"

48. Which statement with regard to suicide is correct?
    A. Suicidal intent is a sign of a serious physical health problem.
    B. More women commit suicide than men.
    C. Men use less violent means than women to commit suicide.
    D. Suicide is a common cause of death among adolescents.

49. Which is a common warning signal for suicidal intent?
    A. Giving away prized possessions
    B. Extreme suspiciousness
    C. Extreme interest in a dangerous sport
    D. Performing well in school

50. When working with clients who have a distorted perception of reality, the support worker will generally be most effective if he or she:
    A. Encourages the client to discuss the voices they hear
    B. Tries to reorient the client back to reality
    C. Avoids all unnecessary physical contact
    D. Changes the subject

CHAPTER 35

Confusion, Delirium, and Dementia

TRUE OR FALSE

Circle T for true or F for false.

1. T F Never tell a confused client the date and time.

2. T F When caring for confused clients, you should provide newspapers and magazines and access to television and radio.

3. T F It is all right to rearrange the furniture or belongings of a confused client.

4. T F Delirium is a permanent, persistent mental confusion.

5. T F Delirium is an emergency.

6. T F Repetitive behaviours are usually harmless, and the client can be allowed to continue such actions.

7. T F People with Alzheimer's disease can control their behaviours of forgetfulness, incontinence, agitation, or rudeness if they are shown how.

8. T F Alzheimer's disease progresses slowly at a predictable rate in all people.

9. T F It is important to reason with the cognitively impaired client as a first step when the client is angry and aggressive.

10. T F Considering the behaviour of individuals who have mental illness and cognitive impairment, they are not likely candidates for abuse.

11. T F As a caregiver of clients with cognitive impairment, when entering their personal space, you should approach in an assertive, controlling manner.

12. **T** **F** Delirium is common in younger adults with physical illnesses.

13. **T** **F** The risk of Alzheimer's disease increases after the age of 45.

14. **T** **F** A client with dementia is in danger of having accidents because the client does not recognize safety hazards. Dementia also causes movement and gait problems, increasing the risk of falls.

15. **T** **F** *Catastrophic reaction* refers to a situation in which a person with dementia sees, hears, or feels something that is not real.

16. **T** **F** A caregiver can cause agitation and restlessness by ignoring a client with dementia.

17. **T** **F** When caring for a confused client, face the client and speak clearly and slowly.

18. **T** **F** You should maintain a confused client's routine by following a schedule for meals, bathing, exercise, TV, and other activities.

19. **T** **F** Maintaining a confused client's routine is important because it promotes a sense of order and a familiarity with what to expect.

20. **T** **F** The *sandwich generation* refers to adult children who care for their own children and their parents.

21. **T** **F** Key-code locks are placed at the side of a door to prevent a confused client from wandering.

22. **T** **F** It is ineffective to try to reason with a client with Alzheimer's disease because the client often cannot understand or follow reason.

MULTIPLE RESPONSE

From the list below, choose all of the correct answers.

23. What are the early warning signs of dementia?
    A. Memory loss that affects daily activities
    B. Confusion
    C. Problems finding the right words or following conversations
    D. Poor judgement
    E. Loss of bowel or bladder control
    F. Problems with common tasks
    G. Changes in mood, behaviour, or personality
    H. Loss of interest in activities or hobbies

24. Some of the behaviours associated with early-stage dementia include:
    A. Increase in spontaneity—more outgoing or interested in things
    B. Problems finishing thoughts, following directions, and remembering names
    C. Poor judgement
    D. Blaming others for mistakes, forgetfulness, and other problems
    E. Irritability or defensiveness
    F. Problems performing everyday tasks

25. Ways that caregivers can help to calm a person with dementia who screams include:
    A. Providing a calm, quiet setting
    B. Using touch to calm the client
    C. Playing soft music
    D. Discouraging the client from wearing his hearing aids to reduce noise
    E. Having a family member or favourite caregiver comfort and calm the client

26. How can you help a client with Alzheimer's disease who displays inappropriate sexual behaviour?
    A. Encourage the client's sexual partner to show affection
    B. Send the client to her room
    C. Notify your supervisor if the client repeatedly touches his genitals
    D. Ask the client's family to bring in sex magazines so the client can look at them

27. What are some reasons a family may decide to place a person with Alzheimer's disease in a long-term care facility?
    A. Clients with Alzheimer's disease are not allowed to be in a private home.
    B. Family members cannot meet the person's needs.
    C. Family members have their own health problems.
    D. The person's behaviours present a danger to her or to others.

MULTIPLE CHOICE

Circle the correct answer.

28. How can you maintain the day–night cycle for a confused client?
    A. Keep the room well lit all day and at night
    B. Keep the curtains closed in the client's room all day
    C. Encourage the person to wear regular clothes during the day, not sleepwear
    D. Do not allow the client to be toileted during the night

29. Which statement is true concerning clients with Alzheimer's disease and sundowning?
    A. The client may be frightened by poor light or shadows.
    B. Sundowning occurs only on clear nights when the moon is visible.

C. The client can be talked out of his fears.
D. There is no treatment for sundowning.

30. Interventions that would not help when caring for a client who is confused include:
    A. Stating your name and showing your name tag
    B. Giving very detailed answers to questions to help the client understand
    C. Calling the client by name each time you are in contact with
    D. Encouraging the client to wear his glasses and hearing aid if needed

31. Which of these measures is helpful when a client with Alzheimer's disease is agitated?
    A. Keep the client in a calm, quiet environment.
    B. Complete care very quickly.
    C. Place the client in a darkened room.
    D. Take the client to an area with music, activity, and people.

32. How can a client who wanders be protected?
    A. Making sure the client receives medication to calm him down
    B. Restraining the client to prevent movement or wandering
    C. Going with the client who insists on going outside
    D. Explaining to the client why going outside is not possible

33. Mrs. Burns has Alzheimer's disease. She has been having hallucinations that "kitty cats" are in her closet. What might be helpful?
    A. Distracting her by showing her something else
    B. Explaining to her that there are no cats in the facility she lives in
    C. Asking her to draw a picture of the cat
    D. Turning up the radio

34. When a client suffering with Alzheimer's disease says, "I want to go home," it may be appropriate to answer:
    A. "The weather outside is beautiful today."
    B. "Home is where you are at the present."
    C. "Tell me about your home."
    D. "Let's go for a walk."

35. A broad term describing a progressive deterioration of intellectual function is:
    A. Dementia
    B. Mental illness
    C. Senility
    D. Schizophrenia

36. What guideline should the support worker follow when caring for clients with delirium?
    A. Once clients are on medication, their behaviours will always improve.
    B. It is more important to contain the behaviour than to restrain the behaviour.
    C. Agitated clients should be confronted to assess the problem.
    D. Delirium is never reversible, and the family should be aware of this.

37. When dealing with a client exhibiting aggressive or violent behaviour, the support worker should:
    A. Immediately demand that the client sit down
    B. Approach the client alone so she does not feel threatened
    C. Distract the client by turning the television on
    D. Remain at arms' length at all times

38. What is a classic sign of Alzheimer's disease?
    A. Problems finding or speaking the right word
    B. Repeating statements over and over

C. Engaging in reckless behaviour
D. Forgetting how to perform long division

39. Mr. Parco has Alzheimer's disease. Which of the following is a symptom of this?
    A. Fever
    B. Nausea and vomiting
    C. Cursing or swearing
    D. Alopecia

40. Mr. Janssen tends to wander. Which statement about wandering is true?
    A. There is always a cause.
    B. It is always caused by drug side effects.
    C. Stress and anxiety might be the cause.
    D. The client will eventually get bored and will stop on his own.

FILL IN THE BLANK

Match the signs and symptoms below with the following conditions:

A. *Confusion*
B. *Dementia*

41. _____ May get lost in familiar places

42. _____ Can occur after surgery

43. _____ Anger, restlessness, depression, and irritability may occur

44. _____ May be caused by losses of hearing and sight

45. _____ Progressive loss of cognitive and social functions

Indicate whether each symptom of dementia listed below first occurs in:

A. **Stage 1**
B. **Stage 2**
C. **Stage 3**

46. _____ Restlessness that increases during evening hours

47. _____ Cannot walk or sit

48. _____ Less outgoing and less interested in things

49. _____ Forgets recent events

50. _____ Does not recognize family members

51. _____ May say the same thing over and over again

52. _____ Cannot tell the difference between hot and cold

53. _____ Totally incontinent of urine and feces

54. _____ Disoriented to time and place

55. _____ Cannot communicate

56. _____ Has difficulty following directions

MATCHING

Match the area of concern for people with dementia with its correct care strategy.

57. _____ Follow facility policy for locking doors and windows.

58. _____ Provide plastic eating and drinking utensils.

59. _____ Tell the client that you will provide protection from harm.

60. _____ Give consistent responses.

61. _____ Provide for the client's food and fluid needs.

62. _____ Play music and show movies from the client's past.

63. _____ Make sure the client has eaten, because hunger can increase restlessness.

A. Loss of short-term memory

B. Forgetting a person, place, or time

C. Risk for injury

D. Wandering

E. Sundowning

F. Hallucinations and delusions

G. Reduced ability to meet one's own basic needs

Match the area of concern for people with dementia with a strategy to give care to address that concern.

64. _____ Try bathing the client when he or she is calm.

65. _____ Make sure the client wears an ID bracelet at all times.

66. _____ Approach the client in a calm, quiet manner.

67. _____ Provide a quiet and calm eating environment. Cue chewing behaviours as needed.

68. _____ Ensure the client's eyeglasses and hearing aids are clean and in good repair. Keep area well lit and play soft music.

69. _____ Keep a calendar and clock where the client can see them.

A.   Disorientation to place and time

B.   Displays of aggressive behaviour if startled

C.   Easily distracted during meals

D.   Wandering

E.   Hallucinations and delusions

F.   Fear of personal care

CHAPTER 36

Speech and Language Disorders

TRUE OR FALSE

Circle T for true or F for false.

1. T F Most people with dementia have apraxia.

2. T F Some people with aphasia cannot understand the message.

3. T F People with expressive aphasia are not aware of their mistakes when speaking.

4. T F Dysarthria is caused by weakness in the muscles used for speech.

5. T F Relationships between family members are not affected when someone has a speech disorder.

6. T F Shopping and cooking are not affected when someone has a communication problem.

7. T F Because you do not need to spend time on communication, you can take less time giving care to someone who cannot speak.

8. T F It is a help to the client to finish words for him.

9. T F Use positive statements rather than negative statements.

10. T F Aphasia is seldom permanent.

MULTIPLE RESPONSE

From the list below, choose all of the correct answers.

11. What can cause speech and language challenges?
    A. Genetic problems or conditions present at birth
    B. Poor eating habits
    C. Brain injury, which may be caused by accident, infection, drug abuse, stroke, and so on
    D. Disease
    E. Hearing loss
    F. Brain tumours
    G. Stress incontinence
    H. Problems involving the structures used for speech

12. The basic types of aphasia include:
    A. Receptive aphasia: difficulty speaking or writing
    B. Receptive aphasia: difficulty understanding written or spoken words
    C. Expressive aphasia: difficulty speaking or writing
    D. Motor aphasia: difficulty moving limbs
    E. Expressive–receptive aphasia (also known as global aphasia): difficulty speaking and understanding language

13. Which points describe *dysarthria*?
    A. Clients have difficulty speaking clearly because of weakness or paralysis in the muscles used to speak.
    B. Clients usually have slurred, slow, and soft speech.
    C. Clients often have problems forming words, spacing their words, and breathing while speaking.
    D. Clients cannot move the muscles used to speak.

14. What are some of the emotions people with speech and language disorders may experience?
    A. Frustration
    B. Depression
    C. Anger
    D. Low self-esteem
    E. Excitement
    F. Shame
    G. Guilt

15. How do you provide compassionate care to clients who have speech or language disorders?
    A. Address questions and comments to the client, not to others who are present.
    B. Do not force a client to talk in front of others.
    C. Never show impatience, frustration, or worry when a client is having problems speaking or understanding.
    D. Discourage communication. It will only make the client more angry at herself.
    E. Limit the number of choices to help the client express preferences.

16. How can support workers show their respect for clients with speech or language disorders?
    A. By being encouraging and supportive
    B. By keeping private information confidential
    C. By learning to be comfortable with silence
    D. By taking extra time to explain procedures and not explaining all the steps at once
    E. By speaking slowly and clearly
    F. By being alert to signs the client has not understood you

17. Some guidelines to effective communication with clients with speech or language disorders are:
    A. Minimize distractions by keeping the client alone as much as possible.
    B. Adjust the lighting; make sure the client can see your face clearly and that you can see the client's.
    C. Give the client your full attention; sit next to the client and speak into his ear.
    D. Ask the client questions to which you know the answer; this helps you become familiar with the client's speech.
    E. Determine the subject being discussed; look for non-verbal clues.
    F. Follow the client's lead; change your communication method as needed.
    G. Speak slowly, clearly, and in a normal tone of voice.
    H. Give the client time to respond; do not answer your own questions.
    I. Use simple words and short sentences; focus mainly on action words and words for people, places, and things.
    J. Be patient; repeat yourself as needed.
    K. Use positive statements.
    L. Use appropriate questioning and paraphrasing techniques; ask questions that require only a short answer or shake of the head, and summarize in your own words what the client has said.

M.   Try to speak without the use of gestures or pointing.

N.   Try other communication methods; follow the care plan and use writing and communication boards as needed.

MULTIPLE CHOICE

Circle the correct answer.

18.   Mrs. Ekove can think clearly but cannot speak. Which type of aphasia is she likely to have?
    A.   Expressive aphasia
    B.   Receptive aphasia
    C.   Expressive–receptive aphasia
    D.   Hemiplegia

19.   After asking Mrs. Ekove a question, the support worker should:
    A.   Allow time for the client to process the question
    B.   Expect an answer in a short time
    C.   Repeat the question again immediately
    D.   Ask the client if she is going to answer the question

20.   To ensure that Mr. Ross understands what you have said, you should:
    A.   Always have a witness when you speak to him
    B.   Ask questions to see if he understood you
    C.   Ask him to take notes while you speak
    D.   Not bother to speak; instead, write things down and give him the note

21.   Mrs. Faubert cannot speak. To communicate with her, you should:
    A.   Use body language
    B.   Shout slowly and distinctly
    C.   Use sign language
    D.   Follow the care plan

22.   Communication boards with letters on them would be less useful for:
    A.   Teens who can use e-mail
    B.   An older client who likes to read
    C.   A young adult who is blind
    D.   A school-age child with a tracheostomy

CHAPTER 37

Hearing and Vision Disorders

TRUE OR FALSE

Circle T for true or F for false.

1. **T**   **F**   *Presbyopia* is an age-related change that takes place in the eye.

2. **T**   **F**   Hearing-impaired clients will understand what you are saying if you exaggerate your words.

3. **T**   **F**   *Age-related macular degeneration* is damage to blood vessels in the retina as a result of diabetes.

4. **T**   **F**   Severe vision loss affects a client's physical, social, intellectual, and spiritual health.

5. **T**   **F**   Dogs can be specially trained to work with clients who have hearing loss

6. **T**   **F**   Clients with hearing problems may avoid social situations because they cannot follow conversations.

7. **T**   **F**   Clients with hearing problems sometimes control conversations because they cannot hear if someone else has something to say.

8. **T**   **F**   Clients with hearing problems may get frustrated or irritable as they are under continual stress trying to compensate for their hearing loss.

9. **T**   **F**   If you see a client with a guide dog or a white cane with a red tip , you should recognize that the client is blind.

MULTIPLE RESPONSE

From the list below, choose all of the correct answers.

10. Which of the following guidelines will help you to communicate better with a client with hearing loss?
    A. Alert the client to your presence.
    B. Adjust the lighting so the client can see your face for lip reading.
    C. Increase background noise.
    D. Focus your attention on the client; stand or sit on the side of the unaffected ear, and do not do other tasks while speaking to the client.
    E. Speak in a loud tone of voice; do not shout, and do not cover your mouth when talking.
    F. Check communication aids; make sure the client is wearing hearing aids and eyeglasses, if used.
    G. Adjust your language; state the topic of conversation clearly, and use simple words and short sentences; say things in a different way if the client does not understand you.
    H. Use other communication methods (e.g., use body language or write key words on paper).
    I. Watch for signs of fatigue; avoid tiring the client.

11. What should you do if a hearing aid does not seem to work properly?
    A. Check if the hearing aid is on
    B. Check the battery position
    C. Insert a new battery if needed
    D. Clean the hearing aid with hot soapy water

12. Which are the correct steps to clean an artificial eye?
    A. Wash the eye with mild soap and warm water. Rinse well.
    B. Line a container with a tissue or with toilet paper.
    C. Fill the container with any cleaning solution.
    D. Label the container with the client's name and room number (if in a facility).
    E. Place the container in the drawer in the bedside stand or in another safe place as directed by the client.
    F. Wash the eye socket with hot soapy water. Use a washcloth or gauze square.
    G. Wash the eyelid with mild soap and warm water. Clean from the outer to the inner part of the eye.

13. Which of the following will assist you to care for a client with vision loss?
    A. Adjust the lighting to avoid glare; stand or sit in good light.
    B. Alert the client to your presence; identify yourself when you enter the room, and tell the person when you are leaving the room.
    C. Focus your attention on the client; do not turn or walk away while talking, and do not do other tasks.
    D. Speak in a loud tone; speak slowly and clearly.
    E. Assist with walking.
    F. Assist with eating.
    G. Keep walkways clear and free of clutter.
    H. Keep doors partially opened.

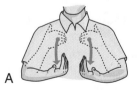 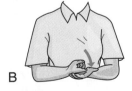

A   B

14. Use the sign language chart in the textbook to identify what signs the client is using in these figures.
    A. Tired
    B. Hungry
    C. Lie down
    D. Get up

MULTIPLE CHOICE

Circle the correct answers.

15. Which disorder may cause vertigo?
    A. Glaucoma
    B. Otitis media
    C. Ménière's disease
    D. Cataracts

16. Which of these signs may indicate a client has a hearing loss?
    A. Speaking very softly
    B. Asking for words to be repeated
    C. Pronouncing words very clearly
    D. Answering questions appropriately while watching television

17. What is the most common cause of blindness in clients over 50?
    A. Cataracts
    B. Age-related macular degeneration
    C. Vertigo
    D. Otitis media

18. Which of these is not a responsibility of a support worker?
    A. Checking the battery position in a hearing aid
    B. Cleaning eyeglasses with warm water
    C. Assisting a client to remove an artificial eye
    D. Removing wax from the ear canal

19. When a client is legally blind, she:
    A. Cannot sense light and has no usable vision
    B. Can sense some light but has no usable vision
    C. Has some usable vision but cannot read newsprint
    D. Sees at 6 metres what a person with normal vision sees at 60 metres

20. What disease do the following statements describe?
    - *In this disease, pressure within the eye is increased.*
    - *It has a gradual or sudden onset.*
    - *The signs and symptoms include tunnel vision, blurred vision, and blue-green halos around lights.*
    - *With a sudden onset, there also is severe eye pain, nausea, and vomiting.*
    A. Ménière's disease
    B. Glaucoma
    C. Cataract
    D. Brain tumour

21. What disease do the following statements describe?
    - *This disease involves increased fluid in the inner ear.*
    - *Symptoms are vertigo, tinnitus, and hearing loss.*
    A. Ménière's disease
    B. Glaucoma
    C. Cataract
    D. Brain tumour

22. What disorder do the following statements describe?
    - *The lens becomes opaque.*
    - *A gradual blurring and dimming of vision occurs.*
    - *It can occur in one or both eyes.*
    - *Aging is the most common cause.*
    A. Ménière's disease
    B. Glaucoma
    C. Cataract
    D. Brain tumour

MATCHING

Match the term related to hearing and vision problems with the correct definition.

23. _____ Dizziness   A.   Otitis media

24. _____ Ringing in the ears   B.   Tinnitus

25. _____ Method of writing using raised dots   C.   Vertigo

26. _____ Infection of the middle ear   D.   Braille

CHAPTER 38

Caring for Mothers and Infants

TRUE OR FALSE

Circle T for true or F for false.

1. **T** **F** Never leave a baby unattended, or with a sibling, in a tub of water.

2. **T** **F** Formula may be heated safely in a microwave.

3. **T** **F** Extra bottles of formula can be stored in the refrigerator and used within 24 hours.

4. **T** **F** Disposable diapers are changed only when the baby has a bowel movement.

5. **T** **F** Disposable diapers can be flushed down the toilet when soiled.

6. **T** **F** The cord stump dries up and falls off in 7 to 10 days.

7. **T** **F** Cord stump care is given every time a bath is given.

8. **T** **F** The diaper is applied loosely while the circumcision is healing.

9. **T** **F** It is important to respond to the cries of the baby or to feed the baby when she is hungry in order to help the baby feel secure and loved.

10. **T** **F** If a baby is "fed on demand," the baby is fed when he asks for food.

11. **T** **F** To reduce the chance of infection, thoroughly rinse bottles and other equipment in cool water.

12. **T** **F** If the baby has had a large bowel movement or has a rash, the genital area should be washed with cool water.

13. **T** **F** When diapering a boy, the cloth diaper is folded in front. For diapering girls, the diaper is folded in back.

14. **T** **F** It is important to plan well when bathing a baby because once you start, you cannot leave the baby.

15. **T   F**   When you are giving a tub bath, the head is washed at the end of the bath.

16. **T   F**   It is important to keep babies' nails short to prevent them from scratching themselves.

17. **T   F**   It is best to trim a baby's nails when he or she is awake so the baby is not frightened.

18. **T   F**   The mother will have an abdominal incision if her baby is delivered by cesarean section.

19. **T   F**   Diarrhea can quickly upset the baby's water balance and harm the baby.

MULTIPLE RESPONSE

From the list below, choose all of the correct answers.

20. When changing a baby on a table or sofa, you can prevent injury by:
    A.   Wrapping a belt around the baby and table top to keep the baby secure
    B.   Keeping one hand on the baby at all times
    C.   Gathering all supplies before beginning the diaper change
    D.   Placing a baby monitor nearby and listening for sounds if you must leave the baby unattended

21. Which health reasons or beliefs would most likely influence parents to choose to have their son circumcised?
    A.   Better hygiene of the genital area
    B.   To possibly prevent certain cancers
    C.   To prevent the foreskin from getting caught in trouser zippers in the future

22. What signs and symptoms would tell you that an infant may be ill?
    A.   Jaundice
    B.   Redness or drainage around the cord stump or circumcision
    C.   Normal temperature
    D.   Limpness and slowness to respond
    E.   Occasional screaming or crying
    F.   Flushed or pale skin
    G.   Heavy perspiration
    H.   Rash
    I.   Soft, rhythmic respirations
    J.   Coughing or sneezing
    K.   Reddened or irritated eyes
    L.   Turning head to one side or putting a hand to one ear (signs of an ear infection)
    M.   Very hungry; eating
    N.   Vomiting most of the feeding or between feedings
    O.   Soft stools
    P.   Stiff neck
    Q.   Signs of dehydration (i.e., fewer than six wet diapers a day, dark yellow urine, decreased saliva and tears, dry lips, dry and wrinkled skin, sunken eyes and top of head)
    R.   Frequent watery, green, mucusy, or foul-smelling stools

23. What ways would be helpful to assist a mother with breastfeeding?
    A.   Wash your hands and remind the mother to wash hers.
    B.   Tell the mother to assume a comfortable position.
    C.   Change the baby's diaper if necessary. Bring the baby to the mother.
    D.   Tell the mother to cover the baby and herself with a blanket.
    E.   Help the mother burp the baby.
    F.   Change the baby's diaper after the feeding if necessary.
    G.   Lay the baby in the mother's bed if the baby is asleep.
    H.   Record what time the baby nursed and how long on each side. Report any problems or concerns.

24. To what types of baby formula must you add water?
    A. Ready-to-feed formula
    B. Powdered formula
    C. Concentrated formula

25. What measures are important to follow for bottlefeeding a baby?
    A. Place the bottle in the microwave to warm up the formula.
    B. Tilt the bottle to check the flow of formula dripping out of the nipple.
    C. Assume a comfortable position for feeding.
    D. Hold the baby close to you.
    E. Tilt the bottle so that the neck of the bottle and the nipple are always filled.
    F. Lay the baby down comfortably and prop up the bottle for the feeding.
    G. Burp the baby after about half the formula and at the end of the feeding.
    H. Keep feeding the baby until all the formula is finished.
    I. Place remaining formula in the refrigerator.
    J. Wash the bottle, cap, and nipple after the feeding.

26. What are good methods for burping a baby?
    A. Hold the baby over your shoulder and gently pat or rub the baby's back.
    B. Support the baby in a sitting position on your lap. Gently pat or rub the baby's back.
    C. If the baby is under 3 months, bounce the baby gently.

27. Cord care includes:
    A. Keeping the cord moist at all times
    B. Washing your hands before and after contact with the umbilical area

    C. Keeping the cord clean by gently wiping around the base of the cord with a cotton ball moistened with warm water
    D. Keeping the top of the diaper below the cord
    E. Reporting any signs of infection (e.g., redness, odour, drainage from the cord)
    F. Giving tub baths until the cord falls off

28. What safety measures should be followed when bathing a baby?
    A. Never leave the baby alone on a table or in the bathtub.
    B. Hold the baby securely throughout the bath.
    C. Keep room temperature between 18 and 20°C.
    D. Water temperature must be between 37.8 and 40.6°C. Measure bath temperature with a thermometer or test with the inside of your wrist.

29. Signs and symptoms of postpartum complications included:
    A. Fever of 38°C or higher
    B. Chills, poor appetite, fatigue, nausea, or vomiting
    C. Lochia that soaks a sanitary pad within 1 hour of application
    D. Foul-smelling lochia
    E. Large number of clots in the lochia
    F. Painful, burning, or difficult urination
    G. Mild abdominal or perineal pain
    H. Bleeding, redness, swelling, or drainage from a cesarean-section incision
    I. Leg pain, tenderness, or swelling
    J. Breast pain, warmth, tenderness, or swelling
    K. Feelings of depression

MULTIPLE CHOICE

Circle the correct answer.

30. Which of these statements is true about cloth diapers?
    A. When soiled, they are placed in the garbage.
    B. They can be easily composted.
    C. They are cheaper to use than disposable diapers.
    D. Cloth diapers are never washed in hot water.

31. How do you remove formula from bottle nipples?
    A. Place them in the sterilizer
    B. Squeeze hot, soapy water through the nipples
    C. Clean them with a bottle brush
    D. Wash them with cool, clean water

32. Which of the following must be reported to the nurse immediately?
    A. The baby "spits up" during burping.
    B. The baby's bowel movement consists of hard, formed stool.
    C. The baby's cord stump is dry.
    D. The baby stops crying when she is picked up and cuddled.

33. A sign of infection in the cord stump would be:
    A. A dried, blackened piece of tissue
    B. Redness or odour at the site
    C. Slight bleeding when the stump falls off
    D. Softening around the base of the cord

34. When a baby boy is circumcised, which of the following is true?
    A. The penis will look red, swollen, and sore.
    B. Urination will be difficult until it is healed.
    C. The area will completely heal in 4 to 6 days.
    D. Circumcision results in shortening the length of the penis.

35. When cleaning the circumcision, what is applied to prevent the penis from sticking to the diaper?
    A. Alcohol
    B. Soap and water
    C. Powder
    D. Petroleum jelly

36. What part of the body is cleaned with cotton swabs during a sponge bath?
    A. Nostrils
    B. Eyes
    C. Ears
    D. No part of the body

37. Which of the following indicates a vaginal or uterine infection in a postpartum woman?
    A. Dark red discharge 3 to 4 days after delivery
    B. An increase in lochia flow with activity
    C. A foul-smelling lochia
    D. Lochia alba that continues for 2 to 6 weeks after delivery

CHAPTER 39

Developmental Disabilities

TRUE OR FALSE

Circle T for true or F for false.

1. T F Mildly affected intellectually disabled people are slow to learn in school.

2. T F People with developmental disabilities do not develop reproductive organs or sexual urges.

3. T F All developmentally disabled people have the same amount of impairment.

4. T F Down syndrome causes some degree of intellectual disability in all affected people.

5. T F Cerebral palsy results from brain damage that occurs during birth.

6. T F Spastic cerebral palsy affects posture, balance, and movement.

7. T F Autism begins in early childhood.

8. T F Autism can be cured with appropriate therapies.

9. T F Children with myelomeningocele may learn to walk using braces or crutches.

10. T F If a child has hydrocephalus, intellectual disabilities and neurological damage will occur without treatment.

11. T F If a mother develops rubella (German measles) during pregnancy, the baby may be intellectually disabled.

12. T F Shaking a baby can cause intellectual disability.

MULTIPLE RESPONSE

From the list below, choose all the correct answers.

13. What are some kinds of developmental disabilities?
    A. Intellectual disabilities
    B. Down syndrome
    C. Autism
    D. Cerebral palsy
    E. Chronic fatigue syndrome
    F. Spina bifida
    G. Fetal alcohol syndrome

14. What are some of the causes of intellectual disability?
    A. Abnormal genes inherited from one or both parents
    B. Missing or extra chromosomes
    C. Illness of mother during pregnancy
    D. Premature birth
    E. Alcohol or drug use during pregnancy
    F. Adequate nutrition
    G. Acquired brain injury

15. The Canadian Association for Community Living believes the following:
    A. Children with an intellectual disability should live with families and be integrated into regular schools whenever possible.
    B. Children with an intellectual disability should learn and play with others who do not have disabilities.
    C. Adults with an intellectual disability should control their own lives to the fullest extent possible.
    D. Adults with an intellectual disability should live in a long-term care facility or have choices and decisions about their care made by others.
    E. People with an intellectual disability have the right to privacy and to love and be loved.
    F. People with an intellectual disability, should learn about sex, sexual abuse, and sexuality issues.

16. What are the physical characteristics of Down syndrome?
    A. Large head
    B. Oval-shaped eyes that slant upward
    C. Flat face
    D. Short, wide neck
    E. Small tongue
    F. Wide, flat nose
    G. Large ears
    H. Short stature
    I. Short, wide hands with stubby fingers
    J. Good muscle tone

17. What therapies will be needed for children and adults with Down syndrome?
    A. Speech therapy
    B. Language therapy
    C. Physical therapy
    D. Occupational therapy

18. Infants at risk for cerebral palsy include those who:
    A. Have a high birth weight
    B. Do not cry in the first 5 minutes after birth
    C. Need mechanical ventilation
    D. Have bleeding in the brain
    E. Have heart, kidney, or spinal cord abnormalities
    F. Have blood problems
    G. Have seizures

19. Lack of oxygen in early childhood can also cause cerebral palsy. The lack of oxygen can occur from:
    A. Near drownings
    B. Choking
    C. Suffocation
    D. Breath-holding
    E. Stroke

20. What impairments may occur with cerebral palsy?
    A. Intellectual disability
    B. Learning disability
    C. Hearing impairments
    D. Speech impairments

E. Vision impairments

F. Bowel and bladder control problems

G. Seizures

H. Attention-deficit hyperactivity disorder

I. Breathing problems

21. What behaviours would you expect to see in a client with autism?
    A. Poor speaking skills
    B. Repeating words or phrases
    C. Starting or maintaining conversation
    D. Repeating body movements
    E. Spending time with others
    F. Showing little reaction to pain
    G. Overreacting to noise and touch
    H. Liking cuddling
    I. Having frequent tantrums for no apparent reason
    J. Forming strong attachment to a single item, idea, activity, or person
    K. Needing routines
    L. Fearing danger
    M. Responding to others
    N. Displaying aggressive or violent behaviour

22. What therapies are used to help the client with autism?
    A. Behaviour modification
    B. Speech and language therapy
    C. Music, auditory, recreation, and sensory therapies
    D. Occupational therapy
    E. Surgical modification
    F. Medication therapy
    G. Diet therapy

MULTIPLE CHOICE

Circle the correct answer.

23. A client with epilepsy:
    A. Can never drive a car
    B. May be able to function normally with medication
    C. Can never get a job
    D. Is intellectually disabled

24. Hydrocephalus is treated by:
    A. Medication
    B. Closing the sac or pouch
    C. Placing a shunt in the brain
    D. Physiotherapy and occupational therapy

25. A client with hemiplegia has a loss of function:
    A. On one side of the body
    B. In corresponding parts on both sides of the body
    C. In all limbs
    D. None of the above

26. A client with cerebral palsy may have:
    A. A large tongue
    B. Short, wide hands
    C. Involuntary movements
    D. A small head

27. A client with autism may:
    A. Show little reaction to pain
    B. Have speech impairments
    C. Have seizures
    D. Drool

MATCHING

Match the types of spina bifida with the correct description.

28. _____   Part of the spinal column is contained in a sac

29. _____   Spinal cord and nerves are usually normal; corrected with surgery

30. _____   Defect in vertebrae closure but cannot be seen on outside of body

31. _____   Pouch contains nerves and spinal cord; loss of function

A.   Spina bifida occulta

B.   Spina bifida cystica

C.   Meningocele

D.   Myelomeningocele

Match the three types of cerebral palsy to the correct muscle movements.

32. _____   Spastic

33. _____   Athetoid

34. _____   Ataxia

A.   Muscle tone is weak, and coordinating movement is difficult.

B.   Movement is stiff and jerky, affecting one or both sides of the body.

C.   Movement is involuntary and involves constant, slow weaving or withering motions in the trunk, arms, hands, legs, and feet.

CHAPTER 40

Assisting With Medications

TRUE OR FALSE

Circle T for true or F for false.

1. **T   F**   An elixir is medication dissolved in a concentrated sugar solution.

2. **T   F**   It is your responsibility to ensure that your clients know about the side effects that can occur when taking their medications.

3. **T   F**   Part of your responsibility is to fill your client's pillbox each week.

4. **T   F**   To make a suppository more comfortable for insertion, apply petroleum jelly to it before handing it to the client.

5. **T   F**   A lozenge is a type of medication.

6. **T   F**   Some medications have to be taken on an empty stomach.

7. **T   F**   It is not within your scope of practice to sign medication administration records (MARs).

8. **T   F**   Medication on transdermal discs is absorbed over 24 hours.

9. **T   F**   You may purchase over-the-counter medications for your client if requested to do so since these are not prescription drugs.

10. **T   F**   Administering medications is beyond your scope of practice.

MULTIPLE RESPONSE

From the list below, choose all of the correct answers.

11. Your role in assisting with medications may involve:
    A.   Reminding the client to take a medication
    B.   Bringing medication containers to the client
    C.   Bringing pre-poured medications, pre-filled syringes, or pillboxes to the client
    D.   Reading the prescription label to the client
    E.   Loosening or removing container lids or opening blister packs

F. Checking the dosage against the medication label
G. Providing water or other fluids as needed
H. Phoning the client's family doctor for prescription refills
I. Supervising the client as she pours the medication into her hand, measuring spoon, or cup

12. A side effect of a medication:
   A. Is a response that occurs along with the main desired response to the medication
   B. May be predictable or unpredictable
   C. Is usually insignificant, so you will not have to look for side effects

13. Which information is contained in most MARs?
   A. The client's name
   B. The client's medication allergies
   C. The name, dose, and administration instructions for each medication
   D. Why the client is taking the medication and what the side effects are
   E. A place to sign or initial after administering the medication

14. Medications should be stored:
   A. In a special place just for the person's medications
   B. In a warm place, such as in a cupboard over the stove
   C. Out of reach of children and of adults with dementia
   D. In the original labelled container, with the lid tightly closed
   E. According to any special storage instructions

15. Some of the "rights" of assisting with medications include:
   A. The right reasons for taking the medication
   B. The right medication

C. The right dose
D. The right route
E. The right time zone
F. The right documentation
G. The right expiration date
H. The right doctor

16. Medications come in many forms. Some examples include:
   A. Ointments; e.g., eye cream
   B. Solids; e.g., aerosols
   C. Syrups; e.g., cough syrup
   D. Drops; e.g., nose drops

17. If the medication is to dissolve under the client's tongue, you should:
   A. Place the medication under the tongue with your fingers
   B. Ask the client to close his or her mouth and let the medication dissolve
   C. Remind the client not to chew or swallow the medication
   D. Provide warm food or fluids to assist in dissolving the medication

18. What information is included on a prescription label?
   A. Pharmacy name
   B. Date filled
   C. Safety warnings for client
   D. Cost of the medication
   E. Physician's name
   F. Number of times the prescription can be refilled
   G. Drug name and dose
   H. Side effects of the medication
   I. Client's name
   J. Client's address

MULTIPLE CHOICE

Circle the correct answer.

19. Mrs. Smythe, one of your clients, is taking an antihistamine and drinking alcohol. What should you do first?
    A. Discuss the situation with your supervisor
    B. Throw away the rest of your client's alcohol
    C. Ask your client if she wants to kill herself
    D. Observe the client for any more drinking

20. You have been assigned to apply Mrs. Smythe's prescription ointment for a rash on her back. What should you do first?
    A. Practise proper hand hygiene
    B. Put on a disposable glove
    C. Wash her skin well and dry it
    D. Check the MAR for the eight rights

21. What is true about transdermal patches?
    A. They have medication that is absorbed through mucous membranes.
    B. They can leak easily, so they need to be covered up with a bandage.
    C. One must be removed before another one can be applied.
    D. They must be rubbed between your hands to activate the medication.

22. What is true about medication suspensions? They:
    A. Are always taken orally
    B. Need to be shaken well before being poured
    C. Usually are dissolved in alcohol
    D. Must be absorbed under the client's tongue

23. Your client cannot open the jar of her aspirin bottle and asks you to do it for her. Should you do this?
    A. Absolutely.
    B. You should tell her that you cannot do this.
    C. You should check with your supervisor first.
    D. You should check the client's care plan first.

24. A dosette is meant to:
    A. Remind clients when to take their medications
    B. Prevent the medication from going stale
    C. Protect the medication from exposure to heat
    D. Keep the medication clean and germ-free

25. A sublingual medication is:
    A. Digested in the client's small intestine
    B. Dissolved in the client's rectum
    C. Absorbed in the client's skin
    D. Dissolved under the client's tongue

26. A metered-dose inhaler is used for:
    A. Medications that are narcotics and under lock and key
    B. Children's medications
    C. Medications that must be inhaled into the lungs
    D. Drug addicts who might overdose easily

27. When working in home care, what should the support worker do with the MAR?
    A. Keep it in her car
    B. Keep it in the client's record at the client's home
    C. Keep it with the support worker's employer
    D. Discard it at the end of each day

MATCHING

Match the abbreviation with the meaning.

28. _____ By mouth   A. bid

29. _____ Per rectum   B. hs

30. _____ Every hour   C. NPO

31. _____ Twice a day   D. PO

32. _____ Every 2 hours   E. qid

33. _____ Four times a day   F. pr

34. _____ Sublingual   G. qd

35. _____ Nothing by mouth   H. qh

36. _____ Hours of sleep   I. q2h

37. _____ Every day   J. sl

Match the medication route with its description.

38. Taken by mouth and swallowed   A. Oral

39. Applied to the skin or mucous membranes   B. Sublingual

40. Breathed in through the mouth or nose   C. Parenteral

41. Placed under the tongue and absorbed into the body   D. Inhalant

42. Injected by a needle into a muscle, a vein, or under the skin   E. Topical

CHAPTER 41

Measuring Height, Weight, and Vital Signs

TRUE OR FALSE

Circle T for true or F for false.

1. **T**   **F**   When you are storing a handheld electronic thermometer, it is placed in a storage box.

2. **T**   **F**   Systole is the period of time the heart muscle is relaxed.

3. **T**   **F**   Bradycardia is a rapid heart rate.

4. **T**   **F**   Blood pressure is normally measured in the brachial artery.

5. **T**   **F**   If you are unsure you have taken an accurate blood pressure reading, you should take off the cuff and try again in 30 to 60 seconds.

6. **T**   **F**   The systolic pressure is the lower pressure.

7. **T**   **F**   Respiratory rates vary with age.

8. **T**   **F**   A tympanic membrane thermometer is inserted into the ear to measure body temperature.

9. **T**   **F**   An axillary temperature taken with a thermometer can take up to 2 minutes to register accurately.

10. **T**   **F**   The earpieces and diaphragm on a stethoscope should never be cleaned with alcohol wipes.

11. **T**   **F**   Rhythm and force are characteristics of a pulse.

12. **T**   **F**   You should avoid using your thumb to take a pulse because you could mistake the pulse in your thumb for the client's pulse.

13. **T   F**   Blood pressure increases with age, up to adulthood.

14. **T   F**   Women usually have higher blood pressures than men.

15. **T   F**   The lower the blood volume, the lower the blood pressure.

16. **T   F**   Stress decreases blood pressure.

17. **T   F**   Blood pressure is higher in overweight people.

18. **T   F**   Blood pressure tends to be lower among people of South Asian, Aboriginal, and African descent.

19. **T   F**   Smoking increases blood pressure.

20. **T   F**   Normal newborn respirations are 30–60 respirations/minute.

21. **T   F**   25–32 respirations/minute is normal for a healthy adult.

MULTIPLE RESPONSE

From the list below, choose all of the correct answers.

22. When would you expect vital signs to be measured?
    A. During physical exams
    B. When a person is admitted to a facility
    C. Once a day for hospital patients
    D. Before and after surgery
    E. Before a fall or other injury
    F. When medications are taken that affect the respiratory or circulatory system
    G. Whenever the client complains of pain, dizziness, light-headedness, shortness of breath, rapid heart rate, or not feeling well
    H. As stated in the care plan (usually daily or weekly)

23. The temperature should not be taken orally if the client:
    A. Is conscious
    B. Has had surgery or an injury to the face, neck, nose, or mouth
    C. Has a nasogastric tube
    D. Is delirious, restless, confused, or disoriented
    E. Is paralyzed on one side of the body
    F. Has a sore mouth
    G. Has a convulsive disorder
    H. Is receiving oxygen therapy

24. Which of the following factors can affect the pulse rate?
    A. Elevated body temperature
    B. Exercise
    C. Pain
    D. Position change
    E. Caffeine
    F. Medications

25. When you are taking a client's blood pressure, which of the following guidelines should you follow?
    A. Take blood pressure on an arm with an IV infusion, cast, or dialysis access site; an injured arm; or on the side where the client has had breast surgery.
    B. Let the client rest for 10 to 20 minutes first.
    C. Measure blood pressure with the client standing.
    D. Use the correct-sized blood pressure cuff.
    E. Apply the cuff over the shirt sleeve.
    F. Make sure the cuff is snug.
    G. Place the diaphragm of the stethoscope firmly over the artery.
    H. Have the manometer clearly visible.
    I. The first sound is the diastolic pressure.
    J. Wait 5–10 seconds before repeating the measurement.

MULTIPLE CHOICE

Circle the correct answer.

26. Why is it important to keep a record of previous vital signs?
    A. The support worker can prove that they were taken.
    B. The doctor or nurse can compare each measurement.
    C. The client's family can check to see if the care is being given.
    D. The support worker can see if the readings obtained are accurate compared with others.

27. When you take the vital signs and they have changed from a previous measurement, what should you do?
    A. Record the results promptly in the client's record.
    B. Circle the changes in red.
    C. Report the changes to the nurse promptly.
    D. Take them again in 15 minutes.

28. Which of these statements about electronic thermometers is not true?
    A. The temperature display is easily read.
    B. If the probe is broken, the client could swallow mercury.
    C. The temperature is rapidly measured.
    D. Disposable covers reduce the possibility of spreading infection.

29. If the client is smoking and you need to take an oral temperature, what should you do?
    A. Provide oral hygiene first.
    B. Wait 15 minutes to take the temperature.
    C. Take a rectal temperature instead.
    D. Wait 45 minutes to take the temperature.

30. For how long should you take an irregular pulse?
    A. 30 seconds
    B. 2 minutes
    C. 5 minutes
    D. 1 full minute

31. When assessing the pulse of a client, which of the following pulse rates should be reported to the nurse immediately?
    A. 72
    B. 50
    C. 60
    D. 98

32. You are assigned to take the blood pressure of several clients. Which of these measurements should you report immediately?
    A. 140/80
    B. 138/90
    C. 150/110
    D. 96/70

FILL IN THE BLANK

Identify whether the following words are used when discussing:

A. *Pulse*
B. *Blood pressure*

33. _____ Radial

34. _____ Bradycardia

35. _____ Hypertension

36. _____ Systole

37. _____ Hypotension

38. _____ Diastole

39. _____ Apical

40. _____ Tachycardia

MATCHING

Match the parts of the stethoscope as indicated in the diagram.

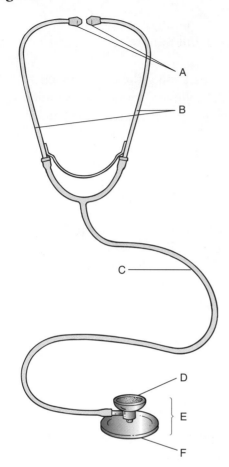

41. _____ Diaphragm

42. _____ Bell

43. _____ Earpieces

44. _____ Binaurals

45. _____ Rubber or plastic tubing

46. _____ Chestpiece

Match the site of the temperature to the normal range for that site.

47. _____ Oral   A. 35.5 to 37.5°C

48. _____ Axillary   B. 34.7 to 37.3°C

49. _____ Tympanic   C. 35.8 to 38.0°C
            membrane

Match the name of the pulse site to where you would find the pulse on the body.

50. Temporal   A. Inside the elbows

51. Carotid   B. Ankles

52. Brachial   C. Top of inner thighs

53. Radial   D. Chest

54. Femoral   E. Sides of the neck

55. Popliteal   F. Knees

56. Dorsalis pedis G. Sides of the head

57. Apical   H. Wrists

Match the normal pulse ranges with the correct age group.

58. 80 to 180   A. 6 to 12 years

59. 70 to 110   B. 2 to 6 years

60. 80 to 120   C. Birth to 1 year

61. 60 to 100   D. 12 years and older

Match the definition with the correct term.

62. Taking the apical and radial pulses at the same time

63. Amount of force exerted against the walls of an artery by the blood

64. Condition in which the systolic blood pressure is below 90 mm Hg and the diastolic pressure is below 60 mm Hg

65. Instrument used to listen to the sounds produced by the heart, lungs, and other body organs

66. A slow heart rate; rate is less than 60 beats per minute

67. Act of breathing air into and out of the lungs

68. Persistent blood pressure measurements above the normal systolic

69. Rapid heart rate; rate is over 100 beats per minute

70. Period of heart muscle relaxation

71. Beat of the heart felt at an artery as a wave of blood passes through the artery

72. Instrument used to measure blood pressure

73. Temperature, pulse, respirations, and blood pressure *(two words)*

74. Period of heart muscle contraction

A. Respiration

B. Tachycardia

C. Apical radial pulse

D. Diastole

E. Hypertension

F. Blood pressure

G. Bradycardia

H. Systole

I. Hypotension

J. Pulse

K. Vital signs

L. Stethoscope

M. Sphygmomanometer

Wound Care

TRUE OR FALSE

Circle T for true or F for false.

1. T F When giving a back massage, massage the bony areas thoroughly.

2. T F Clients sitting in a chair should be reminded to shift their weight every hour.

3. T F When bathing or drying the client, rub vigorously.

4. T F To prevent pressure ulcers, you must frequently check clients who are incontinent to ensure they are not lying on wet linens.

5. T F When applied, adhesive tape should circle the entire body part to prevent swelling.

6. T F Make sure you collect all equipment needed before you begin to change a non-sterile dressing.

7. T F When changing a dressing, you should make sure that the client looks at his or her wound.

8. T F When changing a dressing, you need to wear gloves only if there is drainage.

9. T F You should never apply lotion to a skin crease.

10. T F A stasis ulcer is caused by poor blood return through the veins.

11. T F A skin tear is a very deep cut in the skin.

12. T F Skin tears commonly occur in the head and chest.

13. T F When a lack of blood flow prevents oxygen and nutrients from getting to the cells, skin, and tissues, pressure ulcers occur.

14. T F When a client slides down in a bed or chair, shearing occurs. Blood vessels and tissues are damaged, and blood flow to the area is reduced.

15. T F In obese clients, pressure ulcers can develop where skin surfaces are in contact with each other, causing friction.

16. **T** **F** Heel protectors reduce pressure on the heels by lowering them.

17. **T** **F** A flotation pad or cushion is placed in a pillowcase so the pad does not touch the skin.

18. **T** **F** You should check with the nurse before using soap on a client who is at risk for pressure ulcers because soap can moisturize the skin.

19. **T** **F** Skin should be kept clean and dry and free of moisture from urine, stool, perspiration, and wound drainage.

20. **T** **F** When very small amounts of drainage are expected, a drain is applied to enable the drainage to leave the wound.

21. **T** **F** Scabs and scars are complications of wound healing that are surgical emergencies.

MULTIPLE RESPONSE

From the list below, choose all of the correct answers.

22. Strategies for preventing skin tears include:
    A. Keeping the skin dry and avoiding all moisturizers or skin softeners
    B. Offering fluids
    C. Dressing and undressing the client carefully
    D. Dressing the client in soft clothing with long sleeves and long pants
    E. Keeping your fingernails short and smoothly filed
    F. Keeping the client's fingernails short and smoothly filed
    G. Not wearing rings with raised or large stones

H. Following safety guidelines when lifting and transferring clients
I. Preventing friction and shearing during lifting, moving, transferring, and repositioning (e.g., using a transfer sheet or pad)
J. Avoiding the use of pillows to support arms and legs
K. Being patient and calm when the client resists care
L. Padding bed rails and wheelchair arms, footrests, and leg supports
M. Providing good lighting to help prevent the client from bumping into furniture or walls

23. What are common causes of skin breakdown and pressure ulcers?
    A. Pressure
    B. Age
    C. Friction
    D. Shearing

24. You can prevent shearing and friction by:
    A. Using proper lifting, positioning, and transferring procedures
    B. Never raising the head of the bed more than 30 degrees
    C. Applying a thin layer of cornstarch to the bottom sheets

25. Clients at risk for pressure ulcers are those who:
    A. Are confined to a bed or chair
    B. Require moderate to complete help in moving
    C. Have loss of bowel or bladder control
    D. Have fair to good nutrition
    E. Have altered mental awareness
    F. Have problems sensing pain or pressure
    G. Have circulatory problems
    H. Are younger
    I. Are obese or very thin

26. Why are pillows and blankets used to prevent pressure ulcers?
    A. To prevent skin from being in contact with skin
    B. To reduce moisture and friction between skin surfaces
    C. To keep the client well hydrated

27. Signs that a pressure ulcer is beginning and that therefore should be reported include:
    A. Shivering and a drop in body temperature
    B. An increase in blood pressure
    C. Pale skin
    D. A warm, reddened area

28. Common sites for stasis ulcers are:
    A. Lower legs
    B. Upper arms
    C. Feet
    D. Face and neck

29. What are the risk factors for the development of arterial ulcers?
    A. High blood pressure
    B. Diabetes
    C. Poor diet
    D. Aging
    E. Smoking
    F. Osteoporosis

30. When observing a wound's appearance, what should you continue to monitor?
    A. If the wound is red and swollen
    B. If the area around the wound is warm to the touch
    C. If sutures, staples, or clips are intact or broken
    D. If wound edges are closed or separated, or if the wound has broken open
    E. If the client has complained of the wound getting itchy at times.

31. What are the functions of wound dressings?
    A. They protect wounds from injury and microbes.
    B. They absorb drainage.
    C. They remove dead tissue.
    D. They promote comfort.
    E. They keep the wound warm.
    F. They cover unsightly wounds.
    G. They provide a moist environment for wound healing.
    H. When bleeding is a problem, pressure dressings help control bleeding.

32. How should tape be applied to secure a dressing?
    A. Apply tape to the top, middle, and bottom of the dressing.
    B. Extend the tape several centimetres beyond each side of the dressing.
    C. Place one piece of adhesive tape across the middle of the dressing.

33. What types of tape do not cause allergic reactions?
    A. Paper tape
    B. Plastic tape
    C. Cloth tape

34. If a client has a draining wound, you can help improve the client's appetite by:
    A. Covering the wound with an airtight dressing
    B. Using room deodorizers as directed
    C. Keeping drainage containers out of the client's sight
    D. Telling your supervisor if the client has a preference for certain foods or beverages
    E. Removing soiled dressings promptly from the room

35. How should you remove tape and old dressings from a wound?
    A. Hold the skin down and gently pull the tape toward the wound. Remove adhesive from the skin.
    B. Lift the dressing very gently, and keep the soiled side of the dressing out of the client's sight.
    C. Pull the dressing off as quickly as you can.

36. You can assist a client with a wound by:
    A. Allowing pain medications to take effect before giving care
    B. Ensuring the client stays on complete bed rest until the wound is fully healed
    C. Carefully observing the wound and reporting any signs or symptoms of infection immediately
    D. Practising Standard Practices during all client care

MULTIPLE CHOICE

Circle the correct answer.

37. Which of the following is a cause of skin breakdown?
    A. Good nutrition and hydration
    B. Decreased mobility
    C. Increased circulation
    D. A regular exercise program

38. Which of the following practices are intended to prevent skin tears in clients?
    A. Taking daily baths
    B. Keeping your fingernails short and smoothly filed
    C. Wearing jewellery with large stones
    D. Wearing a clean uniform daily

39. To prevent pressure ulcers, the health care team may place the client on a surface such as:
    A. A firm mattress
    B. A foam, air, alternating air, or gel mattress
    C. Plastic or rubber material
    D. A bed board

40. Which of the following measures are not helpful in preventing pressure ulcers?
    A. Applying moisturizer to dry areas such as hands, elbows, legs, ankles, and heels
    B. Repositioning the client every 4 hours.
    C. Massaging the client well over reddened areas
    D. Keeping the client's heels off the bed.

41. Which of the following measures would help to prevent stasis ulcers?
    A. Making sure the client's clothing fits tightly
    B. Having the client wear elastic stockings as ordered by the doctor
    C. Massaging any reddened area over pressure points
    D. Having the client trim his own toenails weekly

42. Why may pain medication be given before a dressing change?
    A. To reduce discomfort during the dressing change
    B. To prevent the client from looking at the wound
    C. To prevent the client from seeing your non-verbal responses
    D. To prevent contamination of the wound

43. When you are removing an old dressing, it should be:
    A. Shown to the client
    B. Removed quickly from the wound with a quick pull
    C. Removed so that the soiled side is turned away from the client's sight
    D. Placed in the client's garbage can

44. Movement and ambulation can contribute to wound healing by:
    A. Ensuring the wound dressing stays in place
    B. Keeping the client's skin clean and dry
    C. Encouraging better oxygenation of tissue cells
    D. Preventing discoloration of the wound scar

45. Which practice is intended to prevent pressure sores in the client's coccyx area?
    A. Never trimming the client's toenails if the client has diabetes
    B. Brushing the client's teeth, flossing gently, and inspecting the mouth for food particles
    C. Washing bony prominences with gentle soap, rinsing, and drying well.
    D. Encouraging deep breathing and helping the client to cough up phlegm.

46. Clients who are in pain are at greater risk for developing pressure sores because:
    A. They may be more likely to eat and drink well
    B. They cry more and require more emotional support
    C. They are less likely to require pain medication
    D. They are less likely to move and reposition themselves

47. Clients with infected and draining wounds will require more of which two nutrients?
    A. Calcium and iron
    B. Protein and vitamin C
    C. Potassium and phosphorus
    D. Vitamins A and D

MATCHING

Match the type of wound with the correct description.

48. _____ Wound containing large amounts of bacteria

49. _____ Wound that does not heal easily

50. _____ Wound created for therapy

51. _____ Wound resulting from trauma

52. _____ Wound occurring from surgical entry of the urinary, reproductive, respiratory, or gastro-intestinal system

53. _____ Wound that is not infected; microbes have not entered wound

54. _____ Wound in which dermis, epidermis, and subcutaneous tissue are penetrated; muscle and bone may be involved

55. _____ Wound with high risk of infection

56. _____ Wound in which tissues are injured, but the skin is not broken

57. _____ Wound in which skin or mucous membrane is broken

58. _____ Wound in which dermis and epidermis of the skin are broken

A. Persistent wound
B. Clean wound
C. Clean-contaminated wound
D. Closed wound
E. Contaminated wound
F. Dirty (infected) wound
G. Full-thickness wound
H. Intentional wound
I. Open wound
J. Partial-thickness wound
K. Unintentional wound

Match the type of wound drainage with the correct description.

59. _____ Thin, watery drainage that is blood tinged

60. _____ Thick green, yellow, or brown drainage

61. _____ Bloody drainage

62. _____ Clear, watery fluid

A. Purulent drainage

B. Sanguineous drainage

C. Serosanguineous drainage

D. Serous drainage

Match the stage of a pressure ulcer with the correct description.

63. _____ The skin is gone, and underlying tissues are exposed.

64. _____ The skin cracks, blisters, and peels.

65. _____ Drainage is likely.

66. _____ The colour does not return to the skin when pressure is relieved.

A. Stage 1

B. Stage 2

C. Stage 3

D. Stage 4

Match the stage of a pressure ulcer with the correct description.

67. _____ Muscle and bone are exposed and damaged.

68. _____ The skin is red.

69. _____ There may be a shallow crater.

70. _____ The exposed tissue is damaged.

A. Stage 1

B. Stage 2

C. Stage 3

D. Stage 4

Match the phase of wound healing with the correct statement.

71. _____ Tissue cells multiply to repair the wound.

72. _____ The scar eventually becomes thin and pale.

73. _____ Blood supply to the wound increases.

A. Inflammatory phase

B. Proliferative phase

C. Maturation phase

CHAPTER 43

Heat and Cold Applications

TRUE OR FALSE

Circle T for true or F for false.

1. **T   F**   Bags that contain beans or wheat should always be shaken thoroughly before being heated.

2. **T   F**   Applying cold to a body area will constrict blood flow to that area.

3. **T   F**   If the skin is pink, it would be described as being "cyanotic."

4. **T   F**   A *sitz bath* is a warm soak for sore hands and wrists.

5. **T   F**   Support workers can generally apply heat and cold packs to clients.

6. **T   F**   Moist heat usually penetrates more deeply than dry heat.

7. **T   F**   Applying a cold pack for too long can cause the underlying skin to burn.

8. **T   F**   Short-term heat applications affect blood vessels by making them constrict (or become narrow).

9. **T   F**   Heat or cold should be applied at 25-minute intervals.

10. **T   F**   You should check the skin every 15 minutes when moist heat or cold compresses are in place.

11. **T   F**   A *sitz bath* is a type of soak used to clean and soothe perineal or anal wounds.

12. **T   F**   When heat is applied for a long time, blood vessels constrict and therefore blood flow decreases.

MULTIPLE RESPONSE

From the list below, choose all of the correct answers.

13. How does dilation of the blood vessels to an area help in healing?
    A. More blood flows through the vessels and therefore tissues have more oxygen and nutrients for healing.
    B. The dilated blood vessels aid in digestion and make the client feel more relaxed.
    C. Excess fluid and wastes are removed from the area faster, helping to reduce pain and swelling and helping the muscles to relax.

14. Heat applications are used to:
    A. Improve muscle tension
    B. Promote healing
    C. Relieve pain
    D. Reduce tissue swelling
    E. Increase joint stiffness
    F. Improve muscle strength and endurance

15. What people or groups of people are at risk for burns from heat applications?
    A. People with metal implants
    B. Young children
    C. Older adults
    D. Dark-skinned people
    E. People who have decreased sensations (e.g., people with diabetes, spinal cord injuries, or stroke)
    F. People with dementia or confusion
    G. Infants

16. When working in home care, what can you use to apply ice?
    A. Ice bag
    B. Ice collar
    C. Ice cube tray
    D. Ice glove

17. What are the signs of complications when applying heat or cold?
    A. Complaints of discomfort, pain, numbness, or burning
    B. Excessive redness
    C. Blisters
    D. Pink skin
    E. Cyanosis
    F. Shivering

18. What guidelines should be followed for applying heat or cold?
    A. Apply only when ordered by a professional, allowed by your employer, and assigned to do so.
    B. Know how to use the equipment.
    C. Measure the temperature of moist applications after applying.
    D. Follow employer policies for safe temperature ranges.
    E. Do not apply hot applications above 49.1°C.
    F. Ask your supervisor what the temperature of the application should be.
    G. Know the precise site for the application.
    H. Before applying moist heat or cold applications, cover them with a flannel or terrycloth cover, towel, or pillowcase.
    I. Leave at-risk clients unattended only for short periods of time.
    J. Observe the skin for signs of complications. If any signs are observed, immediately remove the application and report to your supervisor.
    K. Observe for changes in the client's behaviour that may indicate sleepiness.
    L. Remind the client not to change the temperature of the application.
    M. Prevent chills. Cover the client with a blanket or robe. Control room drafts.

N. Ask your supervisor how long to leave the application in place. Carefully watch the time.
O. Applications are left on for no more than 25 minutes.
P. Follow Standard Practices.

MULTIPLE CHOICE

Circle the correct answer.

19. Which of these factors may make a client more susceptible to burns?
A. Respiratory disorders
B. Dehydration
C. Circulatory disorders
D. Infections

20. Heat should not be applied to which of these areas?
A. Metal hip and knee replacements
B. Joints
C. Soft tissues
D. Old fractures

21. A sitz bath may cause the client to feel weak or faint because:
A. The bath increases pain in the area.
B. Blood flow increases in the pelvic area, and less blood flows to other body parts.
C. Blood flow decreases in the pelvic area, and more blood flows to other body parts.
D. The client becomes chilled.

22. You applied a commercial cold pack to Jane's ankle as instructed in her care plan. After 3 minutes, she complains of extreme pain to the area. What should you do *first*?
A. Check it after another 2 minutes.
B. Notify your supervisor.
C. Take her pulse in that area.
D. Remove the cold pack.

23. Why are people with thin skin at increased risk for burns with heat and cold applications?
A. They have better circulation than people with thicker skin.
B. They lack enough of a protective adipose layer.
C. They usually have taken better care of their skin.
D. They lack feeling to their skin.

24. Heat and cold applications must be covered before being applied to a client's skin. Which is the best explanation for why this is done?
A. It protects the heat and cold pad from wear and tear.
B. It keeps the heat and cold pack cleaner and free of germs.
C. It helps to prevent contact burns on the client's skin.
D. It prevents skin irritation from the surface of the pack.

MATCHING

Match the types of heat applications with the correct descriptions or statements.

25. _____ A moistened soft pad applied over a body area

26. _____ Does not penetrate deeply

27. _____ Temperature must be lower to prevent injury

28. _____ A warm, moist application that involves immersing a body part in heated water

    A. Dry heat

    B. Moist heat

    C. Compresses

    D. Soaks

Match the types of heat applications with the correct descriptions or statements.

29. _____ The higher temperature needed means burns are still a risk

30. _____ Moist heat is applied to a small area.

31. _____ The water temperature should be hot (36.6° to 41.1°C [97.8° to 105.9°F]).

32. _____ The tub may be used for applying moist heat to a large area.

    A. Dry heat

    B. Moist heat

    C. Compresses

    D. Soaks

CHAPTER 44

Oxygen Needs

TRUE OR FALSE

Circle T for true or F for false.

1. T F The sensor for the pulse oximeter is used only on the fingers.

2. T F The doctor must order oxygen because oxygen is considered a drug.

3. T F The support worker is responsible for administering oxygen.

4. T F The type of device used to deliver oxygen is decided by the nurse.

5. T F You may remove the cannula or mask used to administer oxygen.

6. T F The oxygen flow is turned off when the person receiving oxygen is out of the room.

7. T F Frequent oral hygiene should be given when the client is receiving oxygen therapy.

8. T F Tracheostomy tubes usually consist of three parts.

9. T F A cover is placed over the tracheostomy tube when the client is outside to prevent dust, insects, and other small particles from entering the stoma.

10. T F Suctioning the upper airway may be done through the mouth and pharynx or the nose and pharynx.

11. T F Suctioning the lower airway may be done through the mouth and pharynx or the nose and pharynx.

12. T F Sterile technique is not required for oro-pharyngeal suctioning.

13. T F You may change the settings on a mechanical ventilator as needed.

14. T F When a client has chest tubes, the drainage system is kept above the level of the client's chest.

15. T F Petrolatum gauze is kept at the bedside to cover the insertion site if a chest tube comes out.

16. T   F   Blood must have enough red blood cells because the hemoglobin in the red blood cells picks up oxygen in the lungs and carries it to the cells.

17. T   F   If the client is wearing dark nail polish, you should remove it when you want to use the pulse oximeter.

18. T   F   Gloves are worn to prevent the spread of infection when collecting a sputum specimen because sputum is a bodily fluid.

19. T   F   If you observe that the oxygen rate is not set at the rate the nurse stated, you need to adjust it immediately.

20. T   F   Signs of irritation are evident on the client's arms when he is wearing an oxygen cannula or mask.

21. T   F   A humidifier is often used in oxygen administration to humidify the oxygen so it will not dry the mucous membranes in the client's airway.

22. T   F   Coughing and deep-breathing exercises help to prevent hyperventilation.

MULTIPLE RESPONSE

From the list below, choose all of the correct answers.

23. What processes are involved in the function of the respiratory system ?
    A. Air moves into and out of the lungs.
    B. Carbon dioxide is absorbed into the bloodstream from the lungs.
    C. Oxygen (O_2) and carbon dioxide (CO_2) are exchanged at the alveoli.
    D. The blood transports O_2 to the cells and removes CO_2 from them.

24. What signs and symptoms would tell you the client has hypoxia?
    A. Restlessness
    B. Constipation
    C. Dizziness
    D. Disorientation
    E. Confusion
    F. Behaviour and personality changes
    G. Increased ability to concentrate and follow directions
    H. Apprehension
    I. Anxiety
    J. Fatigue
    K. Agitation
    L. Decreased pulse rate
    M. Decreased rate and depth of respirations
    N. Often leaning forward when in a sitting position
    O. Cyanosis
    P. Dyspnea

25. When a pulse oximeter is used, what should be reported and recorded?
    A. If you think the machine is not working
    B. What the client was doing at the time of the measurement
    C. Oxygen flow rate and the device used
    D. Reason for the measurement (routine or change in the client's condition)
    E. Other observations

26. How is the client instructed to exhale during coughing and deep-breathing exercises?
    A. "Exhale slowly through pursed lips."
    B. "Exhale in short, forceful puffs."
    C. "Exhale until you feel light-headed."
    D. "Exhale until your ribs move as far down as possible."

27. What rules should you follow when handling the tubing for oxygen administration?
    A. Secure connecting tubing (i.e., nasal cannula) in place.
    B. Make sure there are no kinks in the tubing.
    C. Tape or pin the tubing to the client's garment according to employer policy.
    D. Make sure the client does not lie on any part of the tubing.
    E. Never handle the tubing without gloves.

28. What fire safety rules should be followed if oxygen is in use?
    A. Place "No Smoking" signs in the room and on the room door.
    B. Remove materials from the room that ignite easily.
    C. Turn off electrical items before unplugging them.
    D. Use electrical equipment that is in good repair.
    E. Do not use materials that cause static electricity (wool and synthetic fabrics).
    F. Know the location of fire extinguishers and how to use them.
    G. If a fire occurs, turn off the oxygen. Then get the client to safety.
    H. Remind the client and family members about oxygen safety. Report safety hazards immediately.

29. How can you assist the nurse in caring for clients with artificial airways?
    A. By checking vital signs
    B. By observing the client for signs of hypoxia and other respiratory problems
    C. By reporting if an airway comes out or is dislodged
    D. By providing oral hygiene twice a day

30. What are the parts of a tracheostomy tube?
    A. Outer cannula
    B. Middle cannula
    C. Inner cannula
    D. Obturator
    E. Respirator

31. When you are caring for a client with a tracheostomy, you should call the nurse if:
    A. The client shows signs and symptoms of hypoxia
    B. The client shows signs of respiratory distress
    C. The outer cannula comes out
    D. The client must urinate

32. What measures are implemented to prevent aspiration in a client with a tracheostomy?
    A. Make sure dressings do not have loose gauze or lint.
    B. Make sure the stoma or tube is covered at all times.
    C. Make sure the stoma is not covered with plastic, leather, or similar materials.
    D. Instruct the client to take only showers.
    E. Make sure the client is helped with shampooing so that water does not enter the stoma.
    F. Instruct the client that swimming is not allowed.
    G. Make sure the client wears medical alert jewellery and carries a medical alert ID card.

33. What observations should you report to a nurse when assisting with suctioning a client?
    A. An increase in pulse rate
    B. Irregular cardiac rhythms
    C. A drop or rise in blood pressure
    D. Respiratory distress

34. When caring for a client with chest tubes, what information should be observed and reported to the nurse?
    A. Changes in vital signs
    B. Signs and symptoms of hypoxia and respiratory distress
    C. Complaints of pain or difficulty breathing
    D. A decrease in chest drainage
    E. Bubbling in the drainage system increasing, decreasing, or stopping
    F. Any part of the system being loose or disconnected
    G. A chest tube coming out

35. While caring for a client with chest tubes, one of the chest tubes falls out. After you call for help, what should you do next?
    A. Cover the insertion site with sterile petrolatum gauze
    B. Ask the client to hold his or her breath
    C. Keep the client in a supine position
    D. Stay with the client, and then follow the nurse's directions

MULTIPLE CHOICE

Circle the correct answer.

36. A pulse oximeter is used to measure:
    A. The oxygen concentration in arterial blood
    B. The pulse rate
    C. The oxygen concentration in the lungs
    D. The amount of oxygen in the blood

37. Which of these procedures may be done by a support worker?
    A. Administering oxygen therapy
    B. Suctioning
    C. Collecting a sputum specimen
    D. Performing tracheostomy care

38. When is the best time to collect a sputum specimen?
    A. At mealtime
    B. Early in the morning
    C. At bedtime
    D. After using mouthwash

39. What position is often preferred by clients with difficulty breathing?
    A. Lying on one side
    B. Supine position
    C. Orthopneic position
    D. Prone position

40. Which of these statements is true about administering oxygen with a face mask?
    A. It irritates the nose and throat.
    B. It makes talking difficult.
    C. The client may eat and drink while it is in place.
    D. Smoking is allowed in the room where the client is sitting.

41. If the support worker is allowed to set up the oxygen administration system, which of the following would not be allowed?
    A. Connecting the oxygen administration device to the connecting tube
    B. Attaching the flowmeter to the wall outlet
    C. Attaching the humidifier to the bottom of the flowmeter
    D. Applying the oxygen administration device on the person

42. When the nurse is giving tracheostomy care, the support worker may be asked to assist when the ties are removed by:
    A. Holding the inner cannula in place
    B. Cleaning the outer cannula
    C. Cleaning the stoma
    D. Suctioning the tracheostomy

43. Which of the following would be the responsibility of the support worker with a client on a mechanical ventilator?
    A. Resetting the alarm if it rings
    B. Using established hand or eye signals for "yes" and "no"
    C. Listening carefully when the client tells what she needs
    D. Both B and C

44. Mrs. Doronsulic's respiration rate is 34 breaths per minute. This is called:
    A. Eupnea
    B. Bradypnea
    C. Tachypnea
    D. Apnea

45. Which physical condition may *most likely* contribute to Mrs. Tleen's difficulty breathing?
    A. Diabetes
    B. Epilepsy
    C. Iron-deficiency anemia
    D. Glaucoma

46. Narcotic pain medication can affect breathing by causing:
    A. The respiration rate to increase
    B. Thickened mucus in the lungs
    C. Nasal congestion and sinus problems
    D. A suppressed respiration rate and shallower breathing

MATCHING

Match the name of each type of airway with the correct description.

47. An artificial airway inserted through the mouth and into the pharynx

48. An airway inserted through a nostril and into the pharynx

49. An airway inserted through the mouth or nose and into the trachea

50. An airway inserted through a surgical incision into the trachea

A. Tracheostomy tube

B. Endotracheal tube

C. Naso-pharyngeal airway

D. Oro-pharyngeal airway

Match each test with the correct description.

51. _____ Measures the amount of air moving in and out of the lungs

52. _____ Allows the doctor to inspect the trachea and bronchi

53. _____ Punctures and aspirates air or fluid from the pleura

54. _____ Evaluates changes in the lungs

55. _____ Radioactive gas is inhaled, allowing the physician to see what areas are not getting air or blood

56. _____ Laboratory test that measures the amount of oxygen in the blood

A. Chest X-ray

B. Lung scan

C. Bronchoscopy

D. Thoracentesis

E. Pulmonary function tests

F. Arterial blood gases

CHAPTER 45

Assisting With the Physical Examination

TRUE OR FALSE

Circle T for true or F for false.

1. **T** **F** A nasal speculum is used to examine the inside of the nose.

2. **T** **F** The lithotomy position is used to examine a client's breasts.

3. **T** **F** You should always weigh your client before an examination.

4. **T** **F** Sims' position is sometimes used to examine the rectum or vagina.

5. **T** **F** The examiner (either the doctor or the nurse) will take all of the specimens to the laboratory.

6. **T** **F** During a physical examination, only the body part being examined is exposed.

7. **T** **F** The client is asked to urinate before an examination because an empty bladder lets the examiner feel the abdominal organs.

8. **T** **F** When a child is being examined, the parents should leave the room.

MULTIPLE RESPONSE

From the list below, choose all of the correct answers.

9. What should you explain to the client about the positions used in the examination?
   A. Why the position is needed
   B. How to assume the position
   C. How the body is draped for warmth and privacy
   D. What the examiner is looking for
   E. How long the client will stay in the position

MULTIPLE CHOICE

Circle the correct answer.

10. What is a tuning fork used for?
    A. To examine the mouth
    B. To examine the inside of the nose
    C. To examine the internal structures of the eye
    D. To test hearing

11. Which position is the client usually in for an examination of the abdomen?
    A. Lithotomy position
    B. Knee–chest position
    C. Sims' position
    D. Supine position

12. Why does the client need to void before an examination?
    A. To ensure the examiner can feel the abdominal cavity
    B. To ensure a full bladder does not change the normal position and shape of the organs

C. None of the above
D. Both A and B

13. The knee–chest position is used to examine which body part?
    A. Rectum
    B. Abdomen
    C. Breasts
    D. Chest

14. How can you provide your client with privacy during an examination?
    A. Ensure that your client is undressed for the examination
    B. Close the door to the client's room
    C. Let the doctor or nurse explain the examination
    D. Ask everyone to leave the room even if the client has asked for a family member to be present

MATCHING

Match each description with the correct position.

15. _____ Hips down to the edge of the table, knees flexed, feet in stirrups

16. _____ Lying on the side with the upper leg flexed

17. _____ Lying on the back with legs together or knees flexed

18. _____ Kneeling with the body supported on the knees and chest

A. Supine
B. Lithotomy
C. Knee–chest
D. Sims'

Match each instrument name and description with the correct diagram.

19. _____   Ophthalmoscope: used to examine the internal structures of the eye

20. _____   Percussion hammer: used to tap body parts to test reflexes

21. _____   Laryngeal mirror: used to examine mouth, teeth, and throat

22. _____   Tuning fork: used to test hearing

23. _____   Nasal speculum: used to examine the inside of the nose

24. _____   Vaginal speculum: used to open the vagina so it and the cervix can be examined

25. _____   Otoscope: used to examine the external ear and eardrum

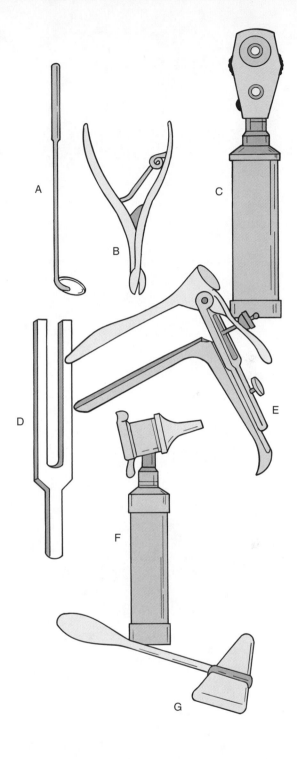

CHAPTER 46

The Client Having Surgery

TRUE OR FALSE

Circle T for true or F for false.

1. **T   F**   The preoperative period may be many days or just a few minutes.

2. **T   F**   Abdominal surgeries do not usually require a preoperative enema.

3. **T   F**   The support worker is responsible for ensuring that the client's chart is in order before the client goes to the operating room.

4. **T   F**   A thrombus can form in the deep leg veins.

5. **T   F**   Elastic stockings help prevent thrombi.

6. **T   F**   The support worker is responsible for telling the client and family about the need for surgery.

7. **T   F**   Behaviours such as crying or being quiet and withdrawn could indicate a client is fearful or concerned about surgery.

8. **T   F**   If the client or family asks you the results of the surgery, you should explain that you cannot provide this information and that you will get your supervisor to help them.

9. **T   F**   To reduce the risk of vomiting and aspiration during anesthesia and after surgery, the client is NPO for 1 to 2 hours before surgery.

10. **T   F**   Children can be prepared for surgery by using anatomical dolls.

11. **T   F**   Some hospitals allow a parent to stay with the child during surgery.

12. **T   F**   Prior to surgery, makeup and nail polish are removed so that the skin, lips, and nail beds can be observed for colour and circulation during and after surgery.

13. **T   F**   Before surgery, you can allow the client to have sips of water during oral hygiene.

14. **T**   **F**   If a client tells you she wants to wear a wedding band or religious medal during surgery, you may secure the item in place with gauze or tape according to hospital policy.

15. **T**   **F**   When a client receives a preoperative medication, he is at risk for falls and accidents.

16. **T**   **F**   The client should be repositioned every 3 to 4 hours after surgery to prevent respiratory and circulatory complications.

17. **T**   **F**   Leg exercises help prevent thrombi.

18. **T**   **F**   Older clients are at higher risk for postoperative respiratory complications.

19. **T**   **F**   After surgery, the client should always dangle the legs prior to ambulating.

20. **T**   **F**   While a client is NPO, fluids can be given by IV therapy.

21. **T**   **F**   Oral hygiene should be provided more frequently while the client is NPO.

22. **T**   **F**   After surgery, if the patient does not void within 2 hours, a catheterization is usually ordered.

23. **T**   **F**   Wound drainage and skin prep solutions can irritate the skin and cause discomfort.

MULTIPLE RESPONSE

From the list below, choose all of the correct answers.

24. Which of the following can you do to assist in the psychological care of the surgical client?
    A.   Listen to the client who voices fears or concerns about surgery.
    B.   Answer any questions about the surgery.
    C.   Explain to the client procedures you will perform and why they are being done.
    D.   Communicate effectively.
    E.   Report to your supervisor verbal and non-verbal signs of client fear or anxiety.
    F.   Report to your supervisor a client's request to see a spiritual advisor.

25. Which of the following are fears the client may have about surgery?
    A.   Disfigurement and scarring
    B.   Disability
    C.   Pain during surgery
    D.   Dying during surgery
    E.   Anesthesia and its effects
    F.   Severe pain or discomfort after surgery
    G.   Tubes, needles, and other equipment used for care

26. Which valuables are removed for safekeeping before surgery?
    A.   Dentures
    B.   Glasses
    C.   Contact lenses
    D.   Lottery tickets
    E.   Hearing aids
    F.   Cash
    G.   Jewellery
    H.   Artificial eyes and prostheses

27. How can you help to protect the client from injury when preoperative medications are given?
    A. Have the client void after medications are given
    B. Refer to the care plan regarding use of side rails
    C. Ambulate the client prior to surgery
    D. Make sure the call bell is within reach
    E. Keep the bed raised to the highest position, regardless of hospital policy

28. What equipment or supplies should be placed in the client's room for use when she returns from surgery?
    A. Thermometer
    B. Stethoscope
    C. Jug of water
    D. Sphygmomanometer
    E. Kidney basin
    F. Tissues
    G. Intake and output record
    H. Intravenous pole
    I. Lunch tray

29. How would you prepare the client's bed and other furniture for his return from surgery?
    A. Make a closed bed
    B. Put the bed in its highest position
    C. Raise the bed rails
    D. Move furniture out of the way for the stretcher

30. Which postoperative observations are important to report to the nurse?
    A. Choking
    B. A drop or rise in blood pressure
    C. Bright red blood from the incision, drainage tubes, or suction tubes
    D. Hypoxia
    E. The need for upper airway suctioning—signalled by tachypnea, dyspnea, moist-sounding respirations, gurgling or gasping, restlessness, or cyanosis
    F. Regular breathing
    G. Weak cough
    H. Complaints of pain or nausea
    I. Vomiting

31. Which complications can be prevented with early ambulation?
    A. Thrombi
    B. Pneumonia
    C. Atelectasis
    D. Pain
    E. Constipation
    F. Emesis
    G. Urinary tract infections

32. Which of the following are factors that can cause pain after surgery?
    A. The extent of the surgery
    B. The incision site
    C. The presence of drainage tubes, casts, or other devices
    D. The age of the client
    E. The gender of the client
    F. Positioning during surgery, which can cause muscle strains and discomfort

MULTIPLE CHOICE

Circle the correct answer.

33. Why is a catheter ordered for some surgeries?
    A. To keep the bladder empty during surgery
    B. To prevent bladder infections postoperatively
    C. To prevent incontinence
    D. So that the client does not have to get out of bed to go to the bathroom

34. Why are coughing and deep-breathing exercises important after surgery?
    A. They prevent pain.
    B. They decrease nausea and vomiting.
    C. They may prevent pneumonia and atelectasis.
    D. They stimulate the circulation.

35. If you want your client to dorsiflex his foot, what movement would you ask him to perform?
    A. Make circles with the toes
    B. Point the toes downward toward the foot of the bed
    C. Point the toes upward as in a standing position
    D. Turn the foot from side to side

36. A general anesthesia produces:
    A. A loss of sensation or feeling in a large area of the body
    B. Unconsciousness and the loss of feeling or sensation
    C. A loss of sensation in a small area
    D. None of the above

37. When a client first returns from the recovery room, the nurse checks the vital signs:
    A. Every 4 hours
    B. Every hour for 4 hours
    C. Every 30 minutes
    D. Every 15 minutes for the first hour

FILL IN THE BLANK

Indicate whether each of the descriptions and examples listed below are associated with:

A. *Elective surgery*
B. *Emergency surgery*
C. *Urgent surgery*

38. _____ Done immediately to save the client's life

39. _____ Done when the coronary arteries are blocked

40. _____ Done for the client's well-being

41. _____ Needed after an accident

42. _____ Must be done soon to prevent further damage or disease

43. _____ Cosmetic surgery, for example

Identify whether each of the events listed below occurs:

A. *Preoperatively*
B. *Postoperatively*

44. _____ A chest X-ray, CBC, and ECG are ordered.

45. _____ Vital signs are measured every 15 minutes for the first hour.

46. _____ Coughing and deep-breathing exercises are performed as ordered.

47. _____ Preoperative teaching is provided.

48. _____ Elastic stockings are applied.

49. _____ An operative permit is signed.

CHAPTER 47

Caring for a Client Who Is Dying

TRUE OR FALSE

Circle T for true or F for false.

1. T F   Many people fear death.

2. T F   During the bargaining stage of grief, the client is usually angry.

3. T F   The client has the right to refuse treatments.

4. T F   As death approaches, body temperature lowers, so the client will need more blankets.

5. T F   Advance directives allow clients to control their future health care.

6. T F   Religious beliefs may help when someone is dying because they can provide comfort.

7. T F   Children under 3 years old have no concept of death.

8. T F   Children 3–5 years of age know that death is final but may not think that it will happen to them.

9. T F   Listening is an important method of communication when dealing with a dying client.

10. T F   Oral hygiene should be given less frequently as death approaches.

11. T F   When death is near, circulation fails and the pulse is fast, weak, and irregular.

12. T F   The goal of palliative care is to relieve pain and suffering while finding a cure.

13. T F   An advance directive is an informal document in which a person states her wishes about future health care, treatment, and personal care.

14. T F   Mucus collecting in the airway that causes wet gurgling sounds is known as the death rattle.

MULTIPLE RESPONSE

From the list below, choose all of the correct answers.

15. How can the support worker help to promote comfort when the dying client has severe pain?
    A. Provide skin care and personal hygiene
    B. Offer back massages
    C. Assist with relaxation techniques
    D. Encourage physical activity
    E. Keep the person in good body alignment

16. What rights are protected in the Dying Person's Bill of Rights?
    A. To be treated as a living human being until death
    B. To maintain a sense of hopefulness
    C. To be cared for by those who can maintain a sense of hopefulness
    D. To express feelings and emotions about one's approaching death
    E. To have decisions about his care made by others
    F. To be free of pain
    G. To die in peace and dignity

17. Some signs of death include the following:
    A. Movement, muscle tone, and sensation are lost.
    B. Peristalsis and other digestive functions slow.
    C. Body temperature drops. Cheyne-Stokes respirations are common.
    D. Pain increases.
    E. The client usually refuses to eat or drink.

MULTIPLE CHOICE

Circle the correct answer.

18. Which of these beliefs about death is common among younger adults?
    A. They may blame themselves when someone dies.
    B. They see death as a reunion with those who have died before them.
    C. They worry about who will care for and support those left behind.
    D. They welcome death as freedom from pain, suffering, and disability.

19. Why are moistened eye pads applied to the eyes of a dying client?
    A. To prevent injury
    B. To shield the eyes from glare
    C. To prevent a darkened room from frightening the client
    D. To relieve discomfort

20. Which of these actions would be helpful to the family of a dying client?
    A. Stay in the room with the family and client as much as possible
    B. Allow family members to give care
    C. Ask the family to leave when visiting hours are over
    D. Ask your clergy member to visit them

21. Which of a client's rights is violated if a health care worker avoids the dying client?
    A. Right to privacy
    B. Right to confidentiality
    C. Right to be free from abuse, mistreatment, and neglect
    D. Right to protection of personal possessions

22. If a client has a "do not resuscitate" order, what action is appropriate when the client dies?
    A. Begin CPR immediately.
    B. The nurse in charge decides if a code should be called.
    C. The support worker may begin CPR if her own beliefs are opposed to taking no action.
    D. No attempt will be made to resuscitate the client.

23. What is a sign that death is near?
    A. The respiratory system fails.
    B. The body temperature falls.
    C. The pulse rate slows.
    D. Pain increases.

24. Which group of clients has fewer fears about death?
    A. Younger adults
    B. Children
    C. Older adults
    D. Middle-aged adults

25. Which is one of the last functions lost?
    A. Taste
    B. Smell
    C. Hearing
    D. Sight

26. Postmortem care includes:
    A. Repositioning the body
    B. Bathing the body
    C. Removing tubes
    D. All of the above

27. A hospice provides:
    A. Palliative care
    B. Active medical care
    C. Care postoperatively
    D. Preoperative care

MATCHING

Match the correct stage of grief with each statement.

28. _____ The client cannot deal with any problem or decision about his illness.

29. _____ The client may wish to talk about people and things that will be left behind.

30. _____ The client may blame others and be difficult to care for.

31. _____ This stage is done privately and on a spiritual level.

32. _____ The client takes care of unfinished business.

A. Denial
B. Anger
C. Bargaining
D. Depression
E. Acceptance

Match the correct stage of grief with each statement.

33. _____ The client is sad and mourns things that have been lost.

34. _____ The client refuses to believe death is close.

35. _____ The client may carry on this stage in private.

36. _____ The client may blame others for problems.

37. _____ This is the final stage of grief.

A. Denial

B. Anger

C. Bargaining

D. Depression

E. Acceptance

FILL IN THE BLANK

Recall the Ontario Resident's Bill of Rights (Box 11-2 in Chapter 11) and match the rights of the dying client in long-term care related to the following actions:

A. *To have privacy and confidentiality*
B. *To visit in private with family and friends*
C. *To be free from abuse, mistreatment, and neglect*
D. *To be in a safe and homelike setting*
E. *To maintain personal choice*

38. _____ Restraints are used only if ordered by a doctor.

39. _____ Do not expose the client unnecessarily.

40. _____ Try to keep equipment and supplies out of sight.

41. _____ Some people avoid a dying person because of superstitions and religious beliefs.

42. _____ The client may refuse treatment.

43. _____ The client may want certain photographs and religious items nearby.

44. _____ The client's final moments and cause of death are kept confidential.

45. _____ A roommate may have to leave the room if the client is too weak to visit outside the room.

46. _____ The health care team needs to respect the client's choices to refuse treatment and not to prolong life.

47. _____ The client's personal property is protected from loss or damage before and after death.

CHAPTER 48

Your Job Search

TRUE OR FALSE

Circle T for true or F for false.

1. **T   F**   The lengthier your résumé, the better it is.

2. **T   F**   A *letter of application* is also called a *cover letter*.

3. **T   F**   Your cover letter should be at least two pages long.

4. **T   F**   If you e-mail your letter and résumé, it is a good idea to also deliver a hard copy.

5. **T   F**   Admit to your prospective employer if you have been fired from a previous job.

6. **T   F**   When filling out a job application, you may skip parts that are unimportant to you.

7. **T   F**   Asking people you know about possible jobs at their workplace is not a good way to find a job.

8. **T   F**   An employer is not as concerned about your dependability as she may be about your job skills.

9. **T   F**   If you were fired from a previous job, it is all right to write on a job application that you resigned.

10. **T   F**   When you are being interviewed for a job, it is acceptable to ask about starting salary, work hours, and new employee orientation.

MULTIPLE RESPONSE

From the list below, choose all of the correct answers.

11. Main basic résumé styles include:
    A. Chronological résumé: highlights employment history, starting with the most current employment and working backward
    B. Functional résumé: highlights skills or functions and briefly lists positions held
    C. Achievement résumé: highlights all successes and awards earned

12. As you write your résumé, which questions should you ask yourself?
    A. Is the information relevant?
    B. Have I been completely honest?
    C. Have I expressed myself clearly?
    D. Is my résumé consistent?
    E. Is there anything I can leave out?

13. Sources to help you in your job search include:
    A. Employment advertisements
    B. Flyers found on windshields
    C. The Internet
    D. College career services
    E. Personal contacts

14. Your letter of application should include:
    A. Relevant skills and qualities
    B. Accomplishments
    C. Contests won
    D. A respectful, capable, and professional tone
    E. Your mailing address
    F. Your signature

15. In an interview, what is the employer looking for?
    A. Someone with the educational qualifications for the job
    B. Someone who has the skills necessary to do the job or who is able to learn these skills
    C. Someone to whom clients and coworkers will respond well
    D. Someone who is reliable, responsible, and motivated
    E. Someone who is attractive and personable

16. You can prepare for an interview by:
    A. Writing possible answers on cue cards
    B. Making a good impression—paying attention to your grooming and clothing
    C. Practising—focusing on listening skills, relaxation techniques, and responses to questions
    D. Planning—deciding what you are going to wear and the route you will take to get there, and preparing a fresh copy of your résumé
    E. Preparing possible questions and answers

17. You can do several things during the interview to help you get the job. Some of these are:
    A. Use a firm handshake.
    B. Do not use the interviewer's first name.
    C. Project a confident image.
    D. Listen carefully.
    E. Answer questions rapidly.
    F. Answer questions honestly.
    G. Be honest about your previous job even if it was unpleasant.
    H. Use experiences to support opinions.
    I. Ask the right questions.
    J. Thank the interviewer for his time.

18. Before accepting a job, find out:
    A. If the offer is conditional
    B. If the job begins with a trial period
    C. If the pay offered is negotiable

19. You have had a job interview and are now planning to write a thank-you note to your interviewer. What points should your note include?
    A. You should express your thanks for the interview.
    B. You should show your interest in the position.
    C. You should state your impressions about the interviewer.
    D. You should sign your name.

MULTIPLE CHOICE

Circle the correct answer.

20. When going to an interview, it would be appropriate to:
    A. Have a glass of wine before arriving to relax you
    B. Wear a sweatsuit and athletic shoes to show that you are physically fit and ready to work
    C. Avoid wearing heavy perfume or aftershave lotion
    D. Arrive exactly at the time of the interview so you do not have to wait around in the reception area

21. Mary Saunders has had four jobs in 1 year. She does not list all four jobs when completing a job application. This is:
    A. Fraud
    B. Invasion of privacy
    C. Her personal choice
    D. Poor work ethics

22. You are completing a job application. How many references should you be prepared to give?
    A. One
    B. Two
    C. Three
    D. Four

23. You are in the waiting area before your interview. What should you do?
    A. Text-message your friend on your cellphone
    B. Talk to the receptionist
    C. Sit quietly
    D. File your nails so they look groomed

24. Which type of answer is best in an interview?
    A. "Yes" and "no" answers
    B. Short explanations
    C. Long explanations
    D. Stalling for time before your answers by counting to three

25. After a job interview, you should:
    A. Thank the interviewer
    B. State that you look forward to hearing from the interviewer
    C. Shake the interviewer's hand
    D. Do all of the above

26. You should write a thank-you note:
    A. The day after the interview
    B. The week after the interview
    C. Two weeks after the interview
    D. Only if you think you would like to work for that agency

STUDY NOTES

STUDY NOTES

STUDY NOTES

STUDY NOTES

STUDY NOTES